THE
OSTEOPOROSIS
SOLUTION

THE
OSTEOPOROSIS
SOLUTION

CARL GERMANO, RD, CNS, LDN
with
WILLIAM CABOT, MD
Diplomate, American Board of Orthopedic Surgery
and
LISA TURNER

Foreword by Ronald L. Hoffman, MD

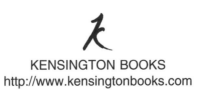

KENSINGTON BOOKS
http://www.kensingtonbooks.com

This book is designed to provide accurate and authoritative information in regard to the subject matter covered. It is sold with the understanding that the publisher is not engaged in rendering medical or related professional services and that without personal consultation the authors cannot and do not render judgment or advice about a particular patient or medical condition. If medical advice is required, the services of a competent professional should be sought. While every attempt has been made to provide accurate information, the author and publisher cannot be held responsible for any errors or omissions.

Baked Kale with Parsnips and Carrots, Southern Style Turnip Greens, Spicy Gingered Greens, Collard and Carrot Raita, and Broccoli Cauliflower Bisque reprinted with permission from *Meals That Heal* by Lisa Turner, published by Healing Arts Press, an imprint of Inner Traditions International, Rochester, VT 05767 Copyright © 1996 by Lisa Turner.

Country Breakfast Scramble, Walnut Pâté, Red Lentil Soup with Arame, Grilled Ginger Cutlets, and Tofu Young, reprinted with permission from *Mostly Macro* by Lisa Turner, published by Healing Arts Press, an imprint of Inner Traditions International, Rochester, VT 05767 Copyright © 1996 by Lisa Turner.

KENSINGTON BOOKS are published by

Kensington Publishing Corp.
850 Third Avenue
New York, NY 10022

Copyright © 1999 by Carl Germano

Library of Congress Card Catalog Number: 98-066722
ISBN 1-57566-391-0

First Printing: January, 1999
10 9 8 7 6 5 4 3 2 1

Printed in the United States of America

ACKNOWLEDGEMENTS

This book is the result of many individuals' hard work and insight. I am indebted to the following colleagues for their significant contributions to this work:

To Rand Skolnick, the man responsible for providing me the opportunity of a lifetime.

To my friend Dr. Ronald L. Hoffman—Medical Director of the Hoffman Center in New York City, host of the syndicated radio program "Health Talk," and author of *Intelligent Medicine*—thank you, Ron, for your kind words and insight in the foreword for this book. During the many years I have known you, your passion, intelligence, and dedication to preventive medicine have been a true inspiration to me.

To my new friend Dr. William Cabot—Diplomate of the American Board of Orthopedic Surgery, President of the William Cabot Group—thank you, Bill, for your outstanding contributions to the chapters on the medical diagnosis of osteoporosis and traditional treatments. Your unflagging enthusiasm and respected experience have made it an honor to have you associated with this book.

To my friend Dr. Jay Lombard—Board-Certified Neurologist and Assistant Clinical Professor of Neurology at Cornell University Medical College, New York Hospital—thank you, Jay, for your tremendous contribution to the bone-immune connection chapter. The respect, admiration, and friendship we share outshines the success of our collaboration on the Brain Wellness Plan.

To my friend Anthony L. Almada, M.Sc.—Nutritional Biochemist and President of IMAGINutrition—thank you, Anthony, for your exemplary contribution to the ipriflavone chapter. I applaud your intellectual accomplishments in product development, and I'm proud to have you associated with this work.

To my friend Brian Appell, B.S., Editor—*ANKH: Perspectives in Health and Well-Being*—Brian, I thank you for your tremendous contribution to writing, editing, and assisting in the preparation of several chapters of this book. Without a doubt, you are a rising star as an editor, writer, and future author.

A SPECIAL ACKNOWLEDGEMENT

To Lisa Turner—writer, editor, author, chef, gardener, friend, and all-around nice person—thank you for the extraordinary job you've done in rewriting this book. From the dry, sterile technical chapters I provided, you've created music, rhythm, and style—your touch is felt on every page. Your lively contribution in the form of the book's recipe section puts the icing on the cake for this book. I am so happy that you are associated with my work and look forward to future collaboration together.

Lastly, I want to thank Paulo Correia and Laura Moutal for their assistance with the illustrations in this book; Lee Heiman for his continued support and assistance; Allan Graubard for his editing of the manuscript; and Paul Dinas, Eileen Bertelli, and others at Kensington for their support of this work.

—Carl Germano, RD, CNS, LDN

DEDICATION

In memory of my father, Joseph. I know you are proud of my accomplishments and I wish you could be here to share them with me. Rest in peace.

To my soul mate, Alise, whose inner wisdom has always provided me with light and direction.

To the blessings in my life, my son Grant and daughter Samantha, who provide the nourishment for my heart and soul.

To my mother, Frances, for your endless love and for always being there.

I love you all.

—CARL GERMANO

To Susie, Brandy, and Adam. You are the source of my happiness.

—WILLIAM CABOT

CONTENTS

FOREWORD

It was with great pleasure that I accepted the invitation of my colleague and good friend Carl Germano to provide an introduction to this book. Carl can always be counted on to dish up cutting-edge information, as he did recently with *The Brain Wellness Plan,* a book I often recommend to my patients with neurological conditions. Carl's commitment to accuracy is reflected in all his writings—there are few individuals in the field of nutrition who possess his energy and originality.

Carl's creativity has been given magnificent support through his twenty-two years in clinical practice and product development in the vitamin and supplement industry. His breakthrough formulations have helped millions of individuals worldwide. It is exciting to see him turn his attention to the problem of bone health because of the magnitude of this problem: more than twenty-five million Americans now have osteoporosis and, with an aging population, the prevalence of this condition is expected to double by the year 2020.

This is where I enter the picture. As a nutritionally oriented physician, I constantly deal with osteoporosis prevention and reversal in my daily practice. In fact, "Keeping Bone Vital" is one of the key chapters in my recent book, *Intelligent Medicine.* In addition, I address numerous calls about osteoporosis on my syndicated radio program, where bone health is a frequent topic.

Recently, I scheduled a show on osteoporosis and found that the station executives got nervous. They asked what kind of demographics I was reaching for, fearing that the topic would be significant only to a limited number of interested elderly people. I explained the prevalence of osteoporosis in other age groups and started the show with that angle. For example, recent studies have shown that teenagers who were given calcium supplements increased bone density by a few percentage points—percentage points that may be crucial for them in later life. Sure enough, the phone lines lit up with calls—and not only from elderly patients, but also from concerned baby boomers, and even from some preventive-minded generation Xers.

You see, osteoporosis has taken on special personal significance for me. After reaching forty-five this year, I came to the shocking realization that the girl who sat in front of me in the first grade, the one whose ponytails I used to pull, may already be well on her way to osteoporosis. Moreover, osteoporosis is not exclusively a female disease. Fully one-third of osteoporosis-related fractures occur in men. While they tend to occur later in men's lives, they are far more deadly in men, whose chance of recovering from hip fractures is half that of women.

In caring for the many patients of my generation who seek my help, I have come to regard osteoporosis as one of the prime preventable diseases in which I can successfully intervene—and by my interventions quite literally alter the course of my patients' lives. Along with heart disease, osteoporosis has taken its place as one of the most preventable medical epidemics of our time. Like heart disease, osteoporosis is a disease of civilization—a product of wrong diet, physical inactivity, and, yes, even stress.

Just as heart disease became recognized as a deadly disease that can strike anyone, osteoporosis has moved from being a once-ignored, silent killer to virtually a national obsession. Millions of women are demanding bone density assessments in the same spirit of prevention that made cholesterol screening an accepted ritual. And while studies cast some doubt on the reliability of elevated cholesterol as a predictor of heart disease susceptibility, decreased bone density is almost certainly a risk for painful, debilitating, and sometimes deadly fractures later in life.

The true quest for medical progress, the altruism of doctors, the concerns of patients, and powerful medical market forces have all converged in the field of osteoporosis detection and treatment, just as they have in the lucrative field of heart disease management. Major drug market strategies for industry blockbusters like Premarin (estrogen replacement therapy), Fosamax, Miacalin, and the recently approved Evista rest on the new public obsession with heading off osteoporosis. Bone densitometry scores are replacing cholesterol-to-HDL ratios as the report cards by which conscientious aging baby boomers gauge their body's health. But the tests are difficult to interpret, even for many doctors, and slight deviations from optimal are increasingly becoming a pretext for drug intervention. Unfortunately, as the potential for long-term consequences of these agents is virtually unknown, we're seeing a rush toward drug therapies for osteoporosis that rivals the recent cholesterol mania.

That's precisely where *The Osteoporosis Solution* can help. Carl Germano, with contributions from Dr. William Cabot, offers us a panoramic view of the problem of bone health. Their concern is not with superficial quick fixes, but with a comprehensive lifetime strategy for staving off osteoporosis. Their approach is predicated on the fact that bone is living tissue, not just a repository for calcium and, as such, is subject to the sum total of influences—both positive and negative—that affect the whole human organism. As an experienced and innovative nutritionist, Carl rejects what I have come to call "the Tums® theory" of osteoporosis prevention espoused by many conventional physicians.

The Tums® theory holds that calcium replacement is the nutritional be-all and end-all of bone health. The theory also assumes that when it comes to calcium, the cheaper the agent used, the better, and that the form of the agent is not important. These arguments fly in the face of scientific evidence that a multitude of agents—vitamins, minerals, essential fatty acids, amino acids, and phytonutrients—play major roles in maintaining bone health, and that calcium bioavailability, which differs according to form and delivery system, impacts absorption and assimilation. All these factors are clearly and elegantly addressed in *The Osteoporosis Solution*.

But the true keystone of *The Osteoporosis Solution* is a nutritional breakthrough that I believe will be one of the most important and lasting to hit the nutrition field in a long time, taking its rightful place among such contenders as glucosamine sulfate, St. Johns Wort, and echinacea. This major player is called ipriflavone, a derivative of the class of compounds called isoflavones naturally found in soy and other plants. In more than sixty human clinical trials, ipriflavone has been shown to increase bone density as well as or better than estrogen replacement therapy or Calcitonin. The ipriflavone story, which Carl elucidates beautifully in *The Osteoporosis Solution,* is highly plausible. We have long known that soy, vegetables, and certain herbs are repositories of countless as-yet unidentified substances that impact human health in heretofore unrecognized ways. Based on the results of the aforementioned human clinical trials, I have now begun incorporating ipriflavone in treating my own osteoporosis patients.

While the ipriflavone story is quite remarkable, Carl presents yet another fascinating factor in osteoporosis: the bone-immune connection. As he did with his colleague Dr. Lombard in their book, *The Brain Wellness Plan,* he shows how the immune system is directly connected with bone, presenting a fascinating and pertinent explanation for every practitioner and osteoporosis patient. They reveal the intimate relationship of the immune system with the skeletal system, and show how it can play both constructive and destructive roles in bone health. Perhaps even more important, they show how nutritional supplements can modulate potentially destructive interactions between the immune and skeletal systems.

The Osteoporosis Solution offers incredible insights regarding ways to maintain healthy bones and treat osteoporosis using a complementary medical/nutritional approach. So enjoy the book, and get set to embark on your personal journey toward optimum bone health.

—*Ronald L. Hoffman, M.D., Medical Director,*
the Hoffman Center, New York City

INTRODUCTION

On the morning of Wednesday, April 13, I picked up my copy of the *New York Times*, settled into my chair, and started reading. The first thing that caught my eye was a feature article entitled "Study Says Thousands Die from Reactions to Medications." The article noted that more than 100,000 people die every year from adverse reactions to medications, making drug reactions one of the leading causes of death in this country.

The response from friends and colleagues was instantaneous and overwhelming. As for me, I didn't quite understand what they were so shocked about. This was old news indeed—annual reports from the Center for Disease Control (CDC) have shown for years that thousands of adverse reactions, including deaths, are attributable to prescription drugs. This fact has been a major impetus in the movement of Americans toward nutritional medicine, vitamin supplements, and complementary health therapies.

During all my years in clinical practice, I have had one primary objective: to get my patients *off* medications via dietary modification and aggressive nutritional supplementation. While I've had much success here, it did not come easily. In fact, twenty years ago I was considered unorthodox in my approach, and my methods raised many eyebrows in the medical institutions for which I worked. Yet, as the patients and their chemistry reports improved, I began to provide the kind of tangible evidence that physicians find so necessary, and rightly so, when encountering a new therapy.

As long as I can remember, I've felt that the real wave of the future in health care involves an integration of the best of both worlds: traditional medicine and complementary, or nutritional, approaches to health care. With that in mind, here are some highlights of what you'll find in this book:

- Ipriflavone—a breakthrough natural treatment for osteoporosis
- The connection between osteoporosis and the immune system
- Dietary influences you should avoid
- The dangerous side effects of commonly prescribed drugs
- Questions you absolutely must ask your doctor
- The best exercises to prevent osteoporosis
- Nutritional supplements—beyond calcium—to build healthy bones

When I began writing this book, I didn't realize how close we are to reaching this new frontier in nutritional medicine, especially with more and more physicians already espousing, or coming to espouse, nutritional therapy. While I'm happy to experience this paradigm shift in medicine, I'm not satisfied yet: we still have a lot of work ahead of us. With *The Osteoporosis Solution,* I intend to draw on some remarkable findings along this new frontier to address a most debilitating disease.

For too long, patients have had to face osteoporosis with only a mediocre arsenal of medical weapons to help them. Traditional doctors who encourage estrogen treatments as *the* answer to treating osteoporosis also may not tell their patients enough about their possible side effects, including cancer. They'll emphasize the importance of calcium in preventing osteoporosis—but they'll completely ignore the other nutrients that play critical roles in the health and maintenance of healthy bone tissue. Meanwhile, the medical establishment continues to ignore significant existing safety-and-efficacy data on nutritional alternatives.

One of these alternatives, and a major focus of this book, is the dietary supplement ipriflavone. Ipriflavone, a derivative of plant estrogens, will revolutionize our approach to treating osteoporosis—as safely and effectively as estrogen but without the cancer-promoting side effects. It's hard to believe, but it's true. Ipriflavone is backed by a wealth of human clinical trials and is considered a safe alternative to other drugs used in treating osteoporosis. It's widely used in Europe as a medication to treat osteoporosis, but it has been totally ignored in the United States as a viable option for treating this disease.

The Osteoporosis Solution represents a convergence of two healing modalities that have been at war for many years—traditional allopathic medicine and nutritional science. In the past, members of both factions have tended to speak *at* each other rather than *to* each other. But when we put egos and agendas aside and combine the knowledge of both, we can better serve the interests of the patient. This was my mission with my first book, *The Brain Wellness Plan,* and so it is with *The Osteoporosis Solution.*

Osteoporosis has taken on a new face—that of a silent killer disease. The trauma associated with complex bone fractures that typically accompany osteoporosis is responsible for millions of injuries and thousands of deaths every year. And osteoporosis is no longer considered a woman's disease: one-third of all cases will occur in men. So get ready to throw away all your old beliefs about osteoporosis—in this book, we're starting from scratch.

In *The Osteoporosis Solution,* you'll find exciting, breakthrough nutritional alternatives to treat and prevent osteoporosis, along with the most up-to-date information on scientific studies. In addition, we'll show you a powerful nutrition protocol that transcends calcium and estrogen. This treatment plan is designed to guide you and your practitioner on the road to an effective and safe course of treatment. And throughout the book, you'll find the necessary tools—everything from dietary supplements and food suggestions to exercise regimens—to allow *you* to take charge of your health.

In Part One, we begin with the basics of how bone tissue develops and maintains itself throughout life. The intricate relationship between two opposing groups of bone cells—those that build bone and those that break down bone—are reviewed. When you understand their function, you'll be able to understand how various drugs and nutritional agents work in treating osteoporosis. This section of the book ends with a revolutionary vision of the relationship between the bones and the immune system.

With the help of numerous well-documented studies from such prestigious medical institutions as Memorial Sloan-Kettering, Rutgers, and Tufts University, I explain the fascinating role our immune system plays in breaking down and building up bone. This chapter will open the door to a whole new view of the function of the immune system and its role in osteoporosis. In short, bone health depends on immune system health. You'll learn how to use new nutritional agents to modulate the immune system as one factor in preventing osteoporosis.

In Part Two, Dr. William Cabot and I lay the foundation for understanding the *traditional* medical approach to osteoporosis. If we are to unite nutrition and medicine, both sides must understand each other—even if they don't always agree. As we try to be objective at all points, we weigh both the pros and cons of the drug therapy currently being offered. We also explain the latest diagnostic procedures—including the most effective X-ray techniques—in detail, so that you'll know exactly what you're facing before you go to the doctor's office.

In Part Three of *The Osteoporosis Solution,* we turn to the exciting new nutritional therapies and complementary treatments to osteoporosis now available. We'll give you detailed dietary specifications, including what you should (and shouldn't) eat, and list nutritional supplements far beyond calcium that have been proven to promote bone health. Of course, we save the best for nearly last, when we introduce ipriflavone, the safe, effective alternative to estrogen without its dangerous side effects. You'll also find a comprehensive list of other nutritional agents and foods you must add to your diet to boost bone health. Finally, we end with delicious, dairy-free bone building recipes contributed by Lisa Turner, author of *Mostly Macro* and *Meals That Heal.*

It's all too clear that a new era has begun. Studies conducted by the leading researchers around the world have led the most informed health care practitioners to this promising conclusion: by using the best of traditional medicine and nutritional science, you *can* prevent and treat osteoporosis—and any other health condition. Good luck in your journey.

—*Carl Germano, R.D., C.N.S., L.D.N.*

PART ONE

ALL
ABOUT
BONES

1

ANATOMY 101: HOW BONES WORK

You probably take your bones for granted—most of us do. We tend to think of bones as static substances that give our bodies a certain shape and are always there when we need them. But the skeletal system is much more than a brittle coat hanger upon which the muscles and skin are draped; rather, our bones are alive and constantly changing and are related to every single system in our bodies.

The skeletal system is the basic foundation of support and protection for all our other biological systems, but it's only when something goes wrong that we really think about it. Our preschool introduction to skeletons, usually in the context of Halloween spooks and graveyard horror tales, may have left us with a slightly skewed impression of this vital system. But far from being a lifeless collection of minerals stuck together, the skeleton is a living, dynamic system, and the bones that compose it are important to every system of the body.

What exactly is bone and what is its role in a biological system? Before we can understand the crippling disease of osteoporosis, we must first answer these questions. So get set for a short biology lesson. Ready?

Bone Structure 101

Did you ever wonder why children, in their rough-and-tumble world, don't break their bones more often—say, on a daily basis? It's because of the unique structure of our bones in our toddler and preschool days. During the first few years of life, bones are not the hardened structures we usually think of. Instead, they are composed of a rubbery substance called **cartilage,** which is flexible

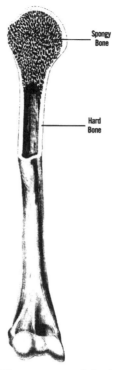

Figure 1-1. The anatomy of the human bone.

and resistant to breaking. As the skeletal system ages, the cartilage is gradually converted to bone through a process called **ossification.** By late adolescence, we have converted cartilage bone to bone bone everywhere but in our ears, where the cartilage remains cartilage.

Even though bone hardens over time, it never really becomes a solid mass of minerals. Instead, its unique structure allows it to be strong yet lightweight. Bone has two primary structural components. The first, **hard bone,** is an outer covering that makes up about 80 percent of the skeletal system. The function of hard bone is to provide protection and support for internal organs and to resist ordinary stresses, like standing and walking. (See Figure 1-1.)

While hard bone is strong, it would soon succumb to breakage from more powerful stresses like running or falling. **Spongy bone,** the second structural component of our skeletal makeup, helps the body compensate for the rigidity of hard bone. Spongy bone, or soft bone, is the internal framework of bone. Because it's porous, it allows flexibility and "give" in response to compression or mechanical stress, effectively acting as a shock absorber. So every time we apply stress to our bones, soft bone absorbs the shock, while hard bone supports our structure.

Making No Bones About Making New Bones

Occasionally, stresses placed on the bones may exceed their capacity to compensate. The result is a break or fracture. But, painful as they are, breaks and fractures aren't permanent. Over time, the bone heals and resumes its original shape, which brings us to the next point:

Bone is a dynamic tissue that is constantly breaking down and reforming.

A unique feature of bone is its ability to grow and adapt to mechanical stress, forming a structure that's best able to resist stress. The basic shape of both hard and soft bone is continually changing as the body redistributes bone material along the points of the greatest or most frequent mechanical stresses. These points, where older bone material may be weaker from constant wear and more prone to possible breakage, are reinforced by the addition of bone material. This ongoing process of replacing old bone with new is greatest during early periods of growth, when bones are assuming their normal shape and contours.

Our bones adapt to mechanical stresses in a unique way, using electrical impulses to detect points of weakness and encourage the addition of bone material along those points.

Bone and Electricity: The Negatives and Positives of Bone Formation

Bones are able to detect their weakest points and deposit bone material to strengthen them through a unique process that uses electrical impulses. Certain crystal-like compounds found in bone have the ability to emit a negative electrical charge when placed under mechanical stress. When the stress is released, a positive charge of equal magnitude is produced. This phenomenon is called **piezoelectricity** and it forms the basis for the theory that electrical charges are the impetus for bone formation and breakdown.

Here's how it works: when a bone is put under stress,

the weakest points tend to bend. They become more concave and emit a negative electrical charge. At the same time, the resulting convex side of the bone generates a positive electrical charge. Through the process of piezoelectricity, these opposing charges stimulate the formation of new bone along the concave side and/or break down existing bone on the convex side. The result is a relative straightening of the bone, making it better able to withstand mechanical stresses.

Over eons of human development, our bones have evolved in such a way as to rely on the stresses of our weight, movement, and even gravity to remain strong and resistant to breakage. Without any mechanical stress at all, our bones would become fragile and weak. In other words, the demands of normal stress are crucial for healthy bones.

To illustrate, let's consider what happens to astronauts in the weightless conditions of outer space. When astronauts are propelled into orbit, they lose considerable amounts of bone mass, since the mechanical stress of gravity is removed and the bones are required to support the body's weight. In the absence of any mechanical stress, the body rids itself of materials used to make bones, and bone mass is consequently lost. When astronauts return to Earth and the subsequent demands of gravity, their bodies respond by making more bone so that their skeletal structures can support their weight in the presence of gravity. And while most of us aren't heading for deep space anytime soon, we're still subject to those same demands of mechanical stress on the bones. Clearly, bone is not a static collection of minerals but a dynamic tissue that's constantly changing. The next question is: what are the compounds in bone that are actually changing?

Collagen: Bone's Superglue

While the *structural* anatomy of bone—both hard and soft—is important in resisting mechanical stress, the *microscopic* anatomy of bone is paramount. Imagine two bridges that are identical in every way except for their composition. One is made of a flexible metal, the other of brittle glass. Even though the two are structurally identical, the glass bridge would soon break because of the material used in its construction. The same applies to bone: even though structure is important, the material used is of primary importance.

We all know the importance of calcium in building bone. But bone relies on far more than calcium to provide strength and support. The only material difference between bone and calcium-rich eggshells, for example, is the presence of proteins that add reinforcement. Without them, our skeletal system would be just as brittle and easy to break as the shell of an egg. These proteins are called collagen, proteoglycans, and glycoproteins.

Collagen is the most abundant protein in the body and is found in most types of **connective tissue**—the cartilage, ligaments, tendons, and bones—that support and hold together other tissue and organs. When collagen is incorporated into connective tissue, it provides resistance to tearing or pulling, while allowing flexibility. Collagen works to reinforce connective tissues, including bones, that are susceptible to tearing or breaking.

A **glycoprotein** is essentially a protein molecule bound to a carbohydrate molecule. **Proteoglycans** are similar to glycoproteins, except that the protein molecule is bound not to one, but to many carbohydrate molecules. The function of proteoglycans is similar to the function of collagen: reinforcing connective tissue. In addition, proteoglycans boost the actions of certain cells that have to do with bone metabolism.

The majority of bone tissue—more than half—is composed of a plethora of minerals, the most abundant being calcium and phosphorus. These two minerals combine into a compound known as **hydroxyapatite,** the substance that forms one of the critical building blocks of bone. The association between hydroxyapatite and collagen cannot be overemphasized:

Without collagen, hydroxyapatite and other minerals cannot combine to form bone.

Getting hydroxyapatite to stick to bone without collagen is something like hanging wallpaper without glue. Collagen is the essential "mortar" that binds together minerals to form bone. The process is like building a brick wall: the first layer—the "cement"—is composed of collagen, proteoglycans, and glycoproteins (the protein substances that add reinforcement). Next comes a layer of hydroxyapatite—the "bricks" that cover the layer of cement. Another layer of "cement" proteins is placed on top of the first, followed by another layer of mineral "bricks." And so it continues.

This process, called **mineralization,** occurs not only in the initial stages of building bone, but throughout life. Collagen and other proteins remain crucial in building bone, just as cement is crucial in building a wall. Without them, all we would have would be a pile of mineral "bricks."

Osteoclasts and Osteoblasts: Bone Breakers and Bone Makers

Even as you read this sentence, millions of cells are eating your bones. It is their intent to chew up and spit out the minerals and collagen that took you weeks to build. This is their sole mission, and nothing will stop them. But at the same time, millions of other cells are rebuilding your bones, reclaiming lost minerals from broken-down bones, and laying down a new foundation of collagen to begin the bone building process again.

Now the question arises: why would these apparently meddlesome little cells keep breaking down and rebuilding bones? Remember that bone isn't static—it's an ever-changing system. As we get older, our bones wear out faster and must be rebuilt to keep our bodies in top condition. This pattern of breaking down and rebuilding to replace old bone with new is termed **remodeling.** It's a delicately balanced procedure: too much formation and the bones become heavy and deformed. Too little, and they become weak and fragile. That delicate balance between breaking down and rebuilding is supervised by a group of specialized cells called **osteoclasts** and **osteoblasts.**

Osteoclasts are the bone *breakers.* It is their responsibility to dismantle the mineral and protein layers that make up bone, a process called **resorption.** Resorption is accomplished when osteoclasts secrete acids and enzymes that break down bone, releasing mineral and protein by-products into the bloodstream. Osteoclasts are believed to be derived from a fusion of cells called **monocytes** that rid the body of foreign invaders and materials by eating them. It is thought that monocytes attach to bone, turn into osteoclasts, and begin the resorption process. (See Figure 1-2.)

Osteoblasts, on the other hand, are the bone *builders.* Without them, our bones would not form normally, if at all. Remember that collagen is the primary essential glue that gives bone reinforcement and flexibility. Osteoblasts synthesize and secrete the protein glue, or **matrix**—collagen, along with proteoglycans and glycoproteins—onto the surface of bone. (See Figure 1-3.)

In the process of producing and secreting matrix, the osteoblast is eventually buried under a layer of collagen and minerals. Remember the brick analogy: think of the osteoblast as the mason who trowels out the cement so the bricks can stick to each other. Suppose

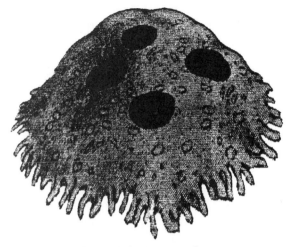

Figure 1-2. An osteoclast.

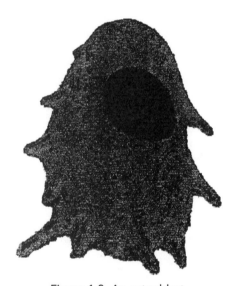

Figure 1-3. An osteoblast.

she builds her brick room without a door, effectively closing herself in. This is essentially what happens to osteoblasts. Once buried, the osteoblast changes into an **osteocyte,** whose job it is to maintain the area of bone that's been constructed.

Both osteoclasts and osteoblasts play a pivotal role in the development, growth, repair, and maintenance of bone. These cells however, have one other equally important function. Osteoclasts and osteoblasts are the gatekeepers for the body's supply of calcium. Without them, blood calcium levels would be impaired—and so would our health.

Bones and the Whole Body

We all know that calcium is a major component of bone. But it also plays a pivotal role in countless everyday functions of the body. When you turned the last page, your brain sent a signal to your hand, and the muscles in your fingers contracted to respond. Without calcium, you couldn't have accomplished even this simple task. Calcium is necessary to keep nerve impulses flowing and allow muscles to contract properly. It's also integral to a number of other body functions, such as blood clotting, hormone regulation, and the initiation of certain metabolic pathways. Your body must have adequate levels of calcium in the blood. Even small imbalances can lead to muscle spasms, anorexia, depression, vomiting, coma, and even death.

Because of calcium's crucial role in the body's functions, the regulation of calcium levels in the blood is a highly specific task that's entrusted to the osteoclasts and osteoblasts. One of the functions of bone is to act as a storehouse for calcium and other minerals. We can take this analogy one step further and think of bone as a bank, with the osteoclasts and osteoblasts functioning as "tellers" who regulate the body's deposits and withdrawals of calcium. In short, if you don't consume enough calcium to provide for basic functions, your body will withdraw calcium from your bone bank to maintain adequate blood levels of calcium and ensure that these functions are carried out.

The body is constantly adjusting the levels of minerals, and especially the level of calcium, in the blood. In order to accomplish this, it must have some form of communication with the osteoclasts and osteoblasts. That's where hormones come in. **Hormones** are a group of chemicals that act as messengers between cells. With the aid of hormones, different cells of the body can communicate with each other. Osteoblasts and osteoclasts are subject to hormonal regulation as well.

The critical point to remember as we go forward is this:

Bone is an integral part of human metabolism, not an isolated mechanical structure, and it affects many bodily systems and functions.

The Bone-Hormone Connection

During childhood and early adolescence, our bones are actively growing, both in length and in thickness. Until young adulthood, our bone formation outpaces bone resorption. This ratio continues until we reach our peak bone mass during our third decade. Then, around the age of forty, our bone resorption begins to exceed formation, and we gradually begin to lose bone mass.

The balance between bone growth and breakdown throughout life depends on the function of certain hormones. These are **estrogen, testosterone, parathyroid hormone, vitamin D,** and **calcitonin.**

Estrogen and Testosterone: Those Sexy Hormones

The hormones that separate the men from the women and the boys from the girls are sex hormones, chiefly **estrogen** in women and **testosterone** in men. Both estrogen and testosterone are derived from cholesterol and affect bone growth throughout our entire lives, but their impact is more pronounced during puberty, when bone growth accelerates. These two hormones increase bone mass by stimulating osteoblast activity. After menopause, a woman's ability to produce estrogen decreases, thereby increasing her risk of developing osteoporosis (see box below). Men, on the other hand, usually produce testosterone throughout their lives and consequently are less likely to suffer from osteoporosis. (There are cases in which testosterone production is hindered, such as in male hypogonadism, a condition marked by the retardation of growth and sexual development. The result is an increased risk of male osteoporosis.)

Researchers have speculated that estrogen may play a greater role than testosterone in bone formation for both women *and* men. Even though men predominantly produce testosterone, they do have the ability to produce estrogen from testosterone. One reason men have higher levels of bone mineralization may be because they can produce estrogen throughout their lives, while women cease to produce estrogen after menopause.

Understanding the Condition:

- **Osteoporosis** is a progressive decrease in bone mass and density, causing skeletal weakness and brittle, fragile bones that are subject to breaking.

> •**Osteopenia** is a reduction of bone mass due to an imbalance between bone breakdown and bone formation. In osteopenia, resorption rates are higher than formation rates, resulting in demineralization and, ultimately, in osteoporosis.
> •**Osteomalacia** is softening of bone in adults caused by a failure of normal bone calcification, primarily as a result of vitamin D deficiency.

Parathyroid Hormone: The Osteoclast's Best Friend

As many as 500 milligrams of calcium are exchanged between the bones and the rest of the body every day. Parathyroid hormone (PTH) is secreted by the parathyroid glands in the neck and plays a major role in the calcium exchange process. If blood calcium levels drop, the parathyroid glands detect this change. In response, they release PTH to alter the activity of bone tissue and the kidneys in a concerted effort to increase blood calcium levels.

The kidneys are responsible for filtering out waste products from the blood, and they also play an important role in blood mineral balance. They do this by acting as gatekeepers for calcium, increasing or decreasing the amount of the mineral excreted in the urine. When PTH is released in response to decreased blood calcium levels, it comes into contact with the kidneys. They, in turn, respond by holding on to calcium, excreting less of it into the urine and returning more to the bloodstream. So, if we're consuming less calcium, the kidneys respond by retaining as much as they can.

PTH also acts on bone by increasing bone breakdown in a somewhat complicated pattern. Osteoclasts, the cells responsible for resorption, or breaking down bone, are not affected by PTH—they just won't listen. Instead, PTH has to communicate indirectly, through osteoblasts, by causing them to produce and secrete a class of proteins called cytokines. **Cytokines** (discussed in detail in the next chapter) are the immune system's chemical messengers and have the capacity to stimulate bone buildup or breakdown.

In essence, it's like the game of telephone we played when we were kids: PTH tells osteoblasts that blood levels of calcium are low. Osteoblasts then tell the osteoclasts to start breaking down bone so that calcium may be released. In other words, PTH increases blood calcium levels in two ways: first, by telling the kidneys to return more calcium to the bloodstream instead of excreting it, and second, by breaking down bone to release calcium.

Vitamin D: Proof That Plants Are People

We have more in common with plants than we may have thought. Even though we're not usually green, humans do share a characteristic with plants in that we, too, can photosynthesize. **Photosynthesis** is the process of making chemical substances under the influence of light. That's how plants make food, and that's how humans make vitamin D. Actually, to call vitamin D a "vitamin" is a misnomer. In reality, vitamin D is a hormone that works with PTH to preserve bone mass.

If our skin is adequately exposed to sunlight, we make enough vitamin D to carry out bodily functions. Vitamin D production becomes a problem when exposure is inadequate through the excessive use of sunscreens or during winter months. A chemical known as **dehydrocholesterol** is responsible for creating vitamin D. In the presence of sunlight, dehydrocholesterol undergoes a series of reactions that result in the formation of vitamin D. But the form produced in the skin isn't biologically active yet—it still has to go through a couple of steps in the kidneys.

As we've already seen, when blood calcium levels drop, PTH is secreted to tell the kidneys to hold on to calcium. PTH also acts on the kidneys to increase the conversion of vitamin D to its active form, **calcitriol.** Calcitriol has the paradoxical effect of both increasing bone breakdown and maintaining bone mass. It does this by affecting the small intestines. Calcitriol helps the body become more efficient at absorbing calcium from our food and supplements. At the same time, it enhances the effects of PTH in breaking down bone. As a result, we're replacing bone that's being broken down with calcium absorbed from the diet. The end result of vitamin D's action is an increase in blood calcium levels while sparing bone mass.

Given the relationship between calcitriol or vitamin D and the digestive system, it's only logical that a deficiency in dietary calcium can lead to decreased deposition and bone mass. When PTH is stimulating bone breakdown and there's not enough calcium being absorbed from the small intestines, the quantity of bone lost will exceed that of bone formed.

Calcitonin: The Yang to PHT's Yin

It's no mistake that *calcitonin* sounds something like *calcium*. In the simplest sense, calcitonin balances the effects of PTH. Just as we have mechanisms to increase calcium blood levels, we must also have mechanisms to decrease calcium blood levels. That's where

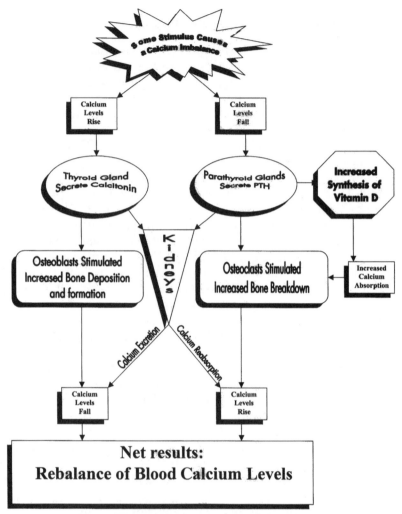

Figure 1-4. Hormonal regulation.

calcitonin comes in. Within the thyroid gland is a group of cells called the **parafollicular cells,** which monitor and respond to increases in blood calcium. Calcitonin acts directly on bone by decreasing osteoclast activity and increasing osteoblast activity. When osteoblast activity is stimulated, the deposit of calcium into bone increases. As calcitonin balances out the effects of PTH on osteoblasts, it also increases the excretion of calcium through the urine. The combined result is increased bone formation and decreased calcium blood levels. (See Figure 1-4.)

What It All Means

If you got a little lost in this chapter, don't worry. Here's the point we're trying to make:

> *Despite its appearance, bone is a dynamic, living tissue that supports human form and function. The delicate balance between osteoclasts that break down bone, osteoblasts that build up bone, and hormones that regulate their activity underscores bone's importance to all the body's systems.*

Because bone is intimately associated with other systems of the body, it is affected by the relative health of those systems. As an example, let's look at two substances we've already talked about: monocytes and cytokines. Both of these are associated with defending the body against harmful organisms and foreign materials, and both play key roles in bone metabolism. Is it possible, then, for aberrations in bone metabolism to occur when the immune system goes awry? In the next chapter, we'll explore this phenomenon and examine the associations between immunity and bone formation and breakdown.

2

THE BONE-IMMUNE CONNECTION

As medicine and the media focus on dramatic diseases and violent killers, osteoporosis—a quiet but deadly disorder—continues to affect millions of lives. More than seventy-five million people worldwide have some form of this progressive and debilitating disorder. The ramifications are far more serious than passing pain or cosmetic inconveniences. Hip fractures that leave patients immobile or bedridden are common, and the risk of hip fracture in older women as a result of osteoporosis is greater than the risk of *all* female cancers combined. And it can be fatal—every year, hundreds of thousands of people die from complications related to osteoporosis.

First, let's look at the simplest definition of this complicated disease:

Osteoporosis is a progressive reduction in bone mass, marked by porous, brittle bones and a greater fragility of bones.

Some of the facts that lead to osteoporosis, like aging, hormonal changes, and nutrition, have long been recognized. Recently, researchers have made another exciting discovery: there is an intimate and crucial relationship between osteoporosis and the immune system. The discovery of this relationship—what I call the **bone-immune connection**—has opened up many new avenues for treating and preventing osteoporosis. In this chapter, we'll look at how the immune system works, examine its intimate relationship with the bones, and look at the nutrients that can enhance this relationship.

The Bone-Immune Connection

When we think of the immune system, we generally visualize busy white blood cells scurrying around protecting our bodies from nasty foreign invaders. Most of us don't think of the immune system as having any relationship to the development of osteoporosis. Even most doctors may not realize the importance of the connection between healthy bones and a strong immune system. But as we saw in the first chapter, our skeletal system is hardly a static, independent structure. Rather, it's a dynamic organism that's intimately related to many other processes and systems in the body. Of these processes and systems, the immune system is one of the most important.

To review: our bones are in a constant process of degradation and restoration. Imagine bone tissue as an architectural landmark, an inherently beautiful structure in partial disarray and in need of constant repair. Various activities take place to support and restore this landmark. Just as parts of a piece of architecture in the process of preservation must be torn down and rebuilt, so must our bones. In our bodies, two groups of cells at the biological construction site—osteoblasts and osteoclasts—are responsible for these tasks.

- **Osteoblasts** are cells involved in *building* bone by creating bone matrix, the mineral and protein compound that makes up bone. They can be compared to the construction workers who mix asphalt and lay concrete for the foundation of the building.
- **Osteoclasts** are cells involved in *breaking down* bone. They're like the workers who operate the jackhammers and pound the asphalt to break down the old building. Their activity disrupts the architecture of bone and ultimately breaks it down.

This process serves two primary purposes: it ensures the maintenance of calcium levels in the body, and it triggers the formation of new bone. Under normal circumstances, a delicate balance is struck between the *buildup* of bone by osteoblasts and the *breakdown* of bone by osteoclasts. **Osteoporosis** can be defined as a disturbance of this delicate balance, resulting in increased activity of osteoclasts and/or decreased activity of osteoblasts. If this imbalance continues, the outcome is a progressive breakdown of bone and the consequent development of osteoporosis. Several factors seem to upset the balance between osteoblast and osteoclast activity. Among these, immunological factors appear to be especially important.

How the Immune System Works

The immune system is one of the most complex systems in our body, and it's related to every other system. It is primarily responsible for protecting us from the harmful effects of bacteria, viruses, and other foreign substances. In carrying out this role, the immune system relies on a highly specialized form of biological communication to coordinate its continuous activity. This communication is accomplished by a group of proteins known as cytokines.

Cytokines are to the immune system what the spoken word is to conversation. They transmit information from cell to cell, stimulating or calming the immune system's activity. And this biological updating isn't confined to the immune system: cytokines are involved in communication between our immune system and all our other organ systems—including the skeletal system. In this fashion, cytokines are able to link seemingly divergent body functions, like bone building and immune functions, in a coordinated and comprehensive manner.

Cytokines are like messengers between the skeletal system and the immune system, and their activity regulates other factors in the development of osteoporosis.

A combination of factors, including low estrogen and progesterone levels and reduced vitamin D and calcium intake, are known to contribute to the development of osteoporosis. What's less commonly recognized, however, is that each of these factors is regulated to some degree by the immune system in general and by cytokines in particular. Cytokines can either promote or prevent osteoporosis. Here's how they interact with hormones, bones, and the immune system.

The Role of Cytokines

Cytokines as a group are divided into two broad categories: **pro-inflammatory agents** and **anti-inflammatory agents.** Cytokines control how long, how fast, and in what part of the body the immune system acts. Their specific message depends on the response needed. In certain sites in the body—for example, an abscessed tooth or swollen glands—cytokines may amplify the immune response, acting as pro-inflammatory agents to fight off foreign invaders. In other sites, cytokines take the role of anti-inflammatory agents, calming immune system activity. While we've been led to believe that the stronger the immune response, the better, this simply isn't true. Like any other process in the body, balance is the key: an overzealous response by the immune system can result in excessive tissue damage.

Certain types of cytokines recently identified by researchers are directly involved in bone metabolism, and consequently, to bone health. Cytokines are related to bone health and osteoporosis in the following ways:

- *They affect the process of bone buildup and breakdown.* Certain types of cytokines influence the activity of osteoblasts and osteoclasts, directing them to break down or build up bone.
- *They are influenced by hormones.* Among the hormones affecting them are estrogen and testosterone, which are known to have an impact on bone health.
- *They are affected by nutritional status and physical activity.* It's widely recognized that nutrient deficiencies—not only of vitamin D and calcium, but also of a range of other important vitamins and minerals—and a sedentary lifestyle are associated with an increased risk of osteoporosis.

Estrogen and Cytokines

The association between estrogen and cytokines as they relate to osteoporosis is especially intriguing. Estrogen deficiency has been closely linked with osteoporosis. Recent studies have also linked the risk of osteoporosis in postmenopausal women with abnormally high levels of a cytokine called **interleukin-1 (IL-1)**.

When women in these studies were treated with estrogen, their bone mass improved, and their blood levels of IL-1 decreased. Interleukin-1 seems to promote bone loss by stimulating the activity of osteoclasts, which break down bone. Estrogen helps to protect bone by reducing IL-1 and keeping osteoclasts in check. In other words: the lower the level of estrogen, the higher the level of interleukin-1, and the higher the level of IL-1, the higher the risk of osteoporosis.

Another type of cytokine, known as **gamma interferon,** is also related to estrogen but in a way that helps build rather than break down bones. Estrogen encourages the action of gamma interferon, which in turn prompts osteoblasts to stimulate bone production. So estrogen plays a duel role in protecting women against osteoporosis:

1. It *discourages* the activity of IL-1 cytokines that stimulate osteo-clasts to break down bone.

2. It *promotes* the activity of gamma interferon cytokines that stimulate osteoblasts to build bone.

The use of estrogen has long been recommended for postmenopausal women to help prevent osteoporosis. But drug therapies using synthetic forms of estrogen can be dangerous and have side effects, such as an increased risk of breast cancer, abnormal uterine bleeding, and breast tenderness and pain. Additionally, estrogen therapy is not appropriate for a significant number of women, especially those at risk of breast and uterine cancers.

But there *are* alternatives to synthetic estrogen. Natural estrogens called **isoflavones** (which we'll talk about in later chapters) are abundant in soy products. One exciting new derivative of isoflavone, called **ipriflavone,** reduces IL-1 activity and helps prevent and treat osteoporosis. (Because ipriflavone represents such a phenomenal breakthrough in the prevention and treatment of osteoporosis, we'll devote an entire chapter to its effects. Please be patient as we mention it throughout the book—you'll get the whole story in Chapter 8.)

Parathyroid Hormone and Interleukin-8

Parathyroid hormone (PTH) is another example of the intricate relationship among osteoporosis, hormones, and the immune system. This hormone is manufactured by the parathyroid glands, a tiny collection of tissue embedded in the thyroid gland at the base of the neck. As we saw in chapter one, PTH is responsible for maintaining adequate blood levels of calcium. When calcium levels falls below a certain level, PTH initiates a process by which calcium is borrowed from the bones and moved into the bloodstream. If your blood calcium level is chronically low, PTH will borrow more and more calcium from the bones, ultimately causing their breakdown. Thus, higher levels of PTH are directly associated with osteoporosis.

An association between PTH and cytokines has also been established. We know that PTH withdraws calcium from bone with the aid of osteoclasts and that it communicates with osteoclasts through the immune system. One type of cytokine known as **interleukin-8 (IL-8)** assists this communication between PTH and osteoclasts, directing them to mobilize calcium from bone.

Vitamin D and Interleukin-1

Vitamin D, which is also classified as a hormone, is another player in the bone–hormone–immune system scenario. Specifically, vitamin D stimulates the formation of bone and plays an invaluable role in preventing osteoporosis. Researchers have long linked vitamin D with healthy bones, but it was originally believed that vitamin D helped fight osteoporosis by increasing calcium absorption. New data have shown that vitamin D works by directly influencing the immune system, which in turn affects bone growth.

Immune system cells are equipped with vitamin D receptors. These little receptors act like cellular satellite dishes: they increase communication between vitamin D and the immune system. Vitamin D affects the action of certain pro-inflammatory cytokines—those that step up the immune response—reducing their action and thereby calming the immune response. Why is this important? In the case of **autoimmune diseases,** the body's immune system goes awry and is misdirected against various sites in the body (see the box below). Because it helps to calm the immune response, certain forms of vitamin D may be useful in combating autoimmune diseases. The connection is this: in some research circles, osteoporosis is thought to be a type of autoimmune disease.

When the Immune System Treats Allies as Enemies

Autoimmune diseases occur when immune activity is mistakenly directed against various regions of our bodies. Lupus and rheumatoid arthritis are two vivid examples of these devastating diseases. The immune system can be compared to a surveillance system. It's responsible for identifying foreign invaders coming in for an attack. Sometimes those invaders are disguised as allies, confusing surveillance efforts. In such cases, the immune system may mistakenly provoke an attack on its own allies instead. This scenario, in which the immune system erroneously wages battle against its own troops, is characteristic of an autoimmune response.

Here's why some researchers suggest that osteoporosis is an autoimmune disorder. Cytokines in the immune system may begin breaking down bone inappropriately if the body can't differentiate between allies and foreign invaders. Vitamin D seems to play a role in treating autoimmune diseases by virtue of its anti-inflammatory properties. Recent research indicates that vitamin D works by inhibiting the actions of interleukin-1. **Interleukin-12 (IL-12)** is thought to play a key role in the development of many autoimmune diseases, and vitamin D has been shown to inhibit the production of IL-12.

As a result, vitamin D *reduces* the damaging effects of cytokines on bone and protects against osteoporosis by virtue of its anti-inflammatory effects.

Other Cytokines

Various other cytokines have also been associated with the breakdown of bone. These include, among others, interleukin-6 (IL-6) and nitric oxide (NO). Understanding the actions of these cytokines can help us understand how to prevent osteoporosis. **Interleukin-6** is a pro-inflammatory cytokine—that is, it increases the activity of the immune system and can cause tissue damage from excessive inflammation—linked to osteoporosis. In addition, IL-6 (like IL-1) promotes osteoporosis by stimulating the activity of osteoclasts. A recent study found that postmenopausal women with higher IL-6 levels showed a corresponding decrease in bone mass. Researchers proposed that one of the beneficial effects of estrogen is its ability to reduce IL-6. Furthermore, certain compounds found in soy and some other foods are *natural alternatives* to estrogen, and as such inhibit IL-6 in activity.

Nitric oxide (NO) functions as a neurotransmitter in our nervous and immune systems, carrying chemical messages between cells. Nitric oxide is normally released by macrophages during periods of inflammation or infection. **Macrophages** are like foot soldiers of the immune system that migrate to the site of battle for hand-to-hand combat. Nitric oxide is a gas and can be compared to a chemical weapon used by macrophages in their battle.

Nitric oxide appears to have a dual role in bone metabolism: in low concentrations, it has been shown to inhibit the bone breaking action of osteoclasts. In other words, small amounts of nitric oxide are necessary to prevent osteoporosis by keeping osteoclasts in check while promoting the activity of osteoblasts. Conversely, at higher concentrations—when the immune system is overactive as a result of a heightened immune response—osteoclasts are stimulated to promote bone breakdown. Thus, higher levels of nitric oxide are less desirable from the standpoint of preventing osteoporosis. In either case, nitric oxide appears to play a crucial role in the bone-immune connection.

Ways to naturally regulate nitric oxide activity, with the hopes of preventing and treating osteoporosis, are currently being explored. One example: in a study conducted by Dr. Lester Packer at the University of California at Berkeley, it has been found that the dietary supplement Pycnogenol® which is derived from a special variety of pine bark was shown to significantly decrease nitric oxide production. The findings of this study suggest that Pycnogenol®

may be a useful therapeutic agent in a variety of nitric oxide sensitive disorders. Ipriflavone, the extraordinary new treatment for osteoporosis we mentioned above, also has the effect of decreasing nitric oxide activity, thereby decreasing the activity of bone breaking osteoclasts. (Again, we'll talk in detail about ipriflavone in its own chapter later in this book.)

There are drugs to regulate nitric oxide activity. One of the more popular of them is a class of drugs called biphosphonates, sold under the trade name Fosamax. Researchers believe these drugs work through their effects on the immune system. Biphosphonates reduce the activity of macrophages, the foot soldiers of the immune system that can produce increased levels of nitric oxide. They also reduce the activity of osteoclasts. But even though they may work, these and other drugs have nasty side effects. We'll talk more later about *natural* ways to regulate nitric oxide and other factors that lead to osteoporosis.

Cytokines and Osteoporosis

Cytokines That Promote Osteoporosis

- Interleukin-1 (IL-1)
- Interleukin-6 (IL-6)
- Interleukin-8 (IL-8)
- Interleukin-12 (IL-12)
- Nitric oxide

Cytokines That Prevent Osteoporosis

- Gamma interferon
- Interleukin-4 (IL-4)
- Interleukin-13 (IL-13)

Nutritional Influences on the Bone-Immune Connection

We've talked about how pro-inflammatory cytokines secreted by the immune system have a definitive role in the activity of bone building osteoblasts and bone breaking osteoclasts. The effect of these inflammatory cytokines includes the inhibition of bone formation and an increase in bone breakdown.

Conversely, our immune system is also important in protecting and rebuilding bone. Researchers in Japan have identified two distinct cytokines that appear to *prevent* the onset and progression of osteoporosis: **interleukin-13 (IL-13)** and **interleukin-4 (IL-4)**. These cytokines inhibit the development and progression of osteoporosis by blocking key biochemical effects seen in pro-inflammatory states. This finding provides more support for the theory that natural anti-inflammatory agents may have a potentially beneficial role in treating osteoporosis.

Several important natural plant compounds also help reduce the activity of the inflammatory cytokines. These include standardized curcumin herb extract, standardized boswellin herb extract, quercitin, vitamin E, Pycnogenol®, vitamin D, and Omega-3 fatty acids. Most of these are available at your health food store. While these substances have not been specifically studied for the control of osteoporosis, their influence on the pro-inflammatory cytokines has been shown in animal and culture studies to reduce osteoclast activity—which results in less bone breakdown.

- **Vitamin E** The activity of interleukin-6 (IL-6)—one of the primary cytokines that increases osteoclast activity—is higher when vitamin E is deficient. In other words, low levels of vitamin E increase IL-6, and IL-6 is significantly implicated in osteoporosis.
- **Quercetin** This antioxidant member of the bioflavonoid family has been shown to inhibit the stimulation of the inflammatory IL-8 activity.
- **Curcumin** Standard extracts of this herb (also known as turmeric) contain powerful phytonutrients that have anti-tumor, antioxidant, and anti-inflammatory effects. Studies have shown that curcumin can decrease the activity of inflammatory cytokines, in particular IL-1 and IL-8.
- **Boswellia** Standard extracts of this herb contain phytonutrients called boswellic acids that have powerful anti-inflammatory and anti-arthritic effects. Commonly used in Ayurvedic medicine as an analgesic, the active constituents of Boswellia inhibit the pro-inflammatory prostaglandins.
- **Pycnogenol®** Pycnogenol® is a registered trademark for a complex of flavonoids and organic acids derived from pine bark extract. Aside from its antioxidant activity, Pycnogenol® can also modulate nitric oxide metabolism and prevent the damage that ensues from excess production.
- **Omega-3 Fatty Acids (DHA and EPA)** Omega-3 fatty acids, derived from fish oils or algae, reduce the activity of IL-1 and IL-6. Remember that high levels of both of these cytokines are linked with

osteoporosis. These fatty acids also play important roles in reducing the activity of inflammatory prostaglandins in the body.

- **Vitamin D** Vitamin D helps to increase the absorption of calcium, and it also has potent immune effects in the body. Regarding osteoporosis, vitamin D in its various forms has been shown to inhibit the function of the osteoporosis promoting cytokine, IL-1.

Inflammatory Cytokine Modulator Formula

The following supplements may be used as part of a total nutritional protocol to treat osteoporosis. This part of the regimen is especially important if inflammation or pain is present, or if specific cytokines have been measured and found to be elevated. As an adjunct, this program should accompany the bone building regimens outlined in later chapters.

Twice a day, take the following supplements with food. If you're taking a multivitamin, check the label. It probably already has vitamins D and E, and may have some of the other compounds as well. If so, you can simply cut those out of the following list.

- Vitamin D—200 IU
- Vitamin E—200 IU
- Quercetin—500 mg
- Standardized Curcumin (Turmeric) Extract—600 mg
- Standardized Boswellia Extract—400 mg
- Pycnogenol®—200 mg
- Omega-3 Fatty Acids (fish oils or algae)—1,000 mg

What It All Means

To sum up the main points so far:

Bone tissue is a dynamic organ in a state of constant change between building up and breaking down. The constant breakdown and buildup of bone is mediated by osteoblasts and osteoclasts, which are regulated by cytokines released from the immune system. The connection between bones and the immune systems allows hormonal and dietary factors to influence bone health.

Decreased levels of estrogen, calcium, vitamin D, and PTH are all factors in the development of osteoporosis. These elements affect bone through their influence on the immune system. Cytokines are the bridges that link these seemingly divergent influences. Future therapies to prevent the development of osteoporosis will use what we know about cytokines and the nutrients that can affect their activity to approach this disease from new and more natural angles.

PART TWO

THE TRADITIONAL APPROACH

3

WHEN THINGS GO WRONG: WHO GETS OSTEOPOROSIS AND WHY

We've talked about bones and the skeletal system. We understand how the skeletal system is intimately related to all organs and systems in the body. Normally, the body—including the skeletal system— functions like a well-oiled machine. But what happens when things go wrong? Now it's time to get down to specifics: what is osteoporosis, and who's at risk? Maybe you think that if you drink lots of milk, or you're only thirty-five, or you're a man, you don't need to worry about osteoporosis. Common myths, all, and none of them true. The fact is, *anyone* can get osteoporosis. And even a gallon of milk a day won't stop bone breakdown if all the other factors aren't in place.

More About Osteoporosis

More than one million fractures per year in the United States are thought to be a result of osteoporosis. At the time of this writing, twenty-five million Americans have osteoporosis. Of these, 80 percent are women. The disease is severely debilitating and may be fatal. And the social cost of osteoporosis is staggering: almost $10 billion a year. It's not hard to see why osteoporosis is considered a disease of epidemic proportions.

Caucasian women are in the highest-risk group. Some studies say that as many as 50 percent of today's fifty-year-old Caucasian women will someday experience a fracture as a result of osteoporosis. The three most common sites of fracture are the vertebrae, the wrists, and the hips. Hip fractures alone are responsible for as many as fifty thou-

sand deaths annually, and most women who suffer hip fractures haven't had any symptoms until the fracture occurs.
More than 50 percent of Caucasian women currently over seventy years old will suffer spinal compression, a severely painful collapse of the vertebrae that can cause paralysis, as a direct result of osteoporosis. And osteoporosis substantially increases the risk of death in the elderly within six months of an injury that involves a fracture.

Osteoporosis and Complementary Therapies

One of the most common—and dangerous—myths about osteoporosis is that it doesn't develop until we're in our eighties or older. Not true. Some people develop signs of osteoporosis as early as their midthirties. Compression of the vertebrae, fractures, and other symptoms of weakened bones are common and cumulative. We've all seen women in their midfifties with the beginnings of a rounded back—what is commonly known as a "dowager's hump." This condition is a direct result of osteoporosis.

It has traditionally been assumed by both patient and physician that these developments are an inevitable by-product of aging. Now we know that's absolutely not true. There are many things you can do to prevent the onset of osteoporosis—and we're not talking about prescription medications here. Diet, exercise, and lifestyle changes are the most important factors in preventing and treating osteoporosis. And the most exciting developments in prevention involve natural substances that have no known side effects. (We'll explore these supplements in detail in later chapters.) In short, osteoporosis is *not* inevitable, and there are safe and natural ways to treat it.

Without a doubt, the most effective mode of treating osteoporosis is with complementary medicine. Perhaps your doctor has suggested herbs and supplements to ease insomnia. Perhaps your chiropractor has recommended X rays to better determine why your leg still hurts. These are examples of complementary approaches to medicine. Sophisticated and conscientious health care practitioners recognize that no one system can do it all and are willing to pick and choose the strongest points from each modality.

Complementary medicine is a practice that combines the best of both worlds of health care—traditional and alternative—for a complete system of treatment.

Complementary medicine is a fairly new concept, and it's still catching on. Back in the good old days—in, say, the 1970s—the role of vitamin and mineral supplements in preventing disease was regarded by the medical community with some disdain. The standard literature claimed that we Americans were getting more than enough vitamins and minerals in our regular diets and that supplements were simply not necessary.

As the years went by, however, researchers started pointing out how beneficial supplements were—especially as preventatives for such extremely serious conditions as heart disease and cancer—and doctors started to come around. So times have changed somewhat. The very vitamins that were regarded as superfluous at best are now widely recognized for their role in preventing devastating diseases. Even so, not every orthodox doctor is guaranteed to know about or believe in the role of vitamins and supplements.

That's where complementary therapies come in. The more *you* know about nontraditional ways to treat osteoporosis, the more you can take charge of your own health. Nutritional therapies are proving to be an integral part of any medical care plan.

Osteoporosis Facts and Figures

- More than seventy-five million people worldwide have some form of osteoporosis.
- The risk of hip fracture in older women is greater than the risk of all female cancers combined.
- More than 50 percent of American women currently over seventy years old will suffer spinal compression as a direct result of osteoporosis.
- Osteoporosis substantially increases the risk of death in the elderly within six months of an injury that involves a fracture.
- Early signs of osteoporosis can be found in women in their twenties and thirties.
- Almost two million American men have osteoporosis, and another three million are at risk.
- Nearly one-third of elderly American men will suffer hip fractures as a result of osteoporosis. Of those, a third will die within a year.
- Older men commonly experience fractures of the spine, wrist, and other bones as a result of osteoporosis.

Along with the recognition of the value of supplements has come a steady, albeit often grudging, acceptance of complementary medicine. Finally, in 1997, an editorial in the *Journal of the American Medical Association* stated that the august group had ranked complementary medicine among the top three subjects it wanted to emphasize in 1998. The article said that AMA's journal would be publishing two issues on complementary medicine in the last quarter of 1998, and that articles on complementary treatments would be featured on a regular basis in issues to come.

Clearly, the medical community as a whole is beginning to accept the fact that there are natural ways to prevent deadly diseases, including osteoporosis. The evidence is hard to ignore: numerous scientific, double-blind studies have documented the amazing effects of complementary treatments. At the same time, an explosion of scientific papers on nutrition and supplements has driven public interest to a near fever pitch. As a result, more and more physicians have been forced to familiarize themselves with complementary approaches.

This is not to malign the traditional medical approach—in some areas, like diagnostic procedures and lifesaving emergency care, it's unsurpassed. But only by combining traditional and alternative procedures are we likely to find the most effective approach for treating osteoporosis—and many other diseases. So once you've been diagnosed using traditional medical procedures, you can seek out complementary therapies that offer safe, effective treatments without known side effects. The therapies we'll discuss in this book are focused on complementary treatments that incorporate the best possible ways to treat osteoporosis. But first, let's look at some of the most commonly asked questions about this deadly disease.

Myths and Misconceptions About Osteoporosis

Simply stated, osteoporosis is a loss of bone mass followed by an increased risk of fracture. It's probably the most common bone disease, and it's responsible for a tremendous amount of pain and suffering in our population. But it's entirely preventable with diet, exercise, lifestyle changes, and the new complementary therapies. And it's possible to identify people in high-risk categories and start preventive treatment even earlier to stave off the devastating consequences of osteoporosis.

Risk factors aside, the truth is that anyone can get osteoporosis. Even men. Even young women. And even people who consume a gallon of milk and a roll of Tums® every day. Let's look at some of the most common myths and misconceptions about osteoporosis:

- *I'm too young to get osteoporosis.* Osteoporosis tends to develop silently, with few symptoms, and when it strikes, it strikes quickly. It can begin to develop in women in their twenties and thirties, and it's not unusual for women in their forties to start feeling its effects. Most people remain unaware of the ravaging effects of osteoporosis until it's too late. In most cases, osteoporosis is discovered only after a seemingly minor fall that results in a fractured hip or vertebrae. That's why it's so important to start preventing osteoporosis early.
- *Only women get osteoporosis.* While it's true that most osteoporosis victims are postmenopausal women, men are far from immune. It's estimated that almost two million American men have osteoporosis, and another three million are at risk. Nearly one-third of elderly American men will suffer hip fractures, and of these, a third will die within a year. Older men also commonly experience fractures of the spine, wrist, and other bones as a result of osteoporosis. In short, osteoporosis in men remains shockingly underdiagnosed and unreported. But men, like women, can prevent osteoporosis safely and effectively using natural supplements and complementary practices.
- *I drink lots of milk—I won't get osteoporosis.* This is one of the most long-standing and pervasive myths about osteoporosis. It's true that calcium is important for bones, but calcium is only one of many minerals and substances that affect bone health. And milk isn't necessarily the best source of calcium anyway. We'll look at all the dietary components that affect bones and discuss other ways to get calcium besides milk in later chapters.
- *If I take calcium supplements, I won't get osteoporosis.* Here's another big misconception. Again, calcium is important and can slow bone loss, but it's not the only component in bone health and osteoporosis. If the other important factors aren't in place—including diet, exercise, and lifestyle—all the calcium on the planet won't protect your bones. Another point: just because you're *taking in* lots of calcium doesn't mean you're *absorbing* lots of calcium. Some common foods can actually block calcium absorption, and certain forms of calcium supplements aren't absorbed as well. We'll talk about these in the chapters on dietary influences and nutritional supplements.
- *My mother has osteoporosis, so I'm doomed to have it too.* Yes, it's true that genetics play a big part in the development of osteoporosis. Studies have shown that genetic factors account for more than half

the variation observed in peak bone mass in the general population. For example, daughters of women with osteoporosis were found to have less bone mass in their spines and hips than women the same age whose mothers *didn't* have osteoporosis. This is not to say that if your mother has osteoporosis, so will you. There are many ways to make your bones healthier. We'll talk about these natural therapies throughout this book.

• *I'll know when I have it.* Too many people think they'll deal with osteoporosis when the symptoms start to show. But it's not as simple as taking handfuls of vitamin C when you start to develop signs of a cold. People who have osteoporosis are relatively symptom-free until the disease is in its advanced stages—another reason it's called a silent killer. Even so, it's never too late. The new natural approaches can not only prevent, but actually treat, osteoporosis.

• *If I have osteoporosis, the worst thing that can happen is I'll get a fracture.* Ask anyone who's had one: fractures are far more than mildly inconvenient. They're extraordinarily painful, especially when they occur in the back, and some fractures can be deadly. Up to 50 percent of elderly women who sustain a fractured hip will die as a result of that fracture. It's not the fracture itself that's deadly, of course, but the ensuing medical complications, such as blood clots and cardiovascular problems.

When any kind of tissue—including bone—is broken, blood clots are formed, and in older people they can be dangerous, especially if the clots travel. A hip fracture renders most people immobile, and prolonged bed rest or inactivity is especially harmful for older people. The immobilized body is quickly devastated by a multitude of medical problems, many of which can prove fatal in the geriatric population.

Cultural Differences in Osteoporosis Risk

Culture seems to play a role in a person's risk of developing osteoporosis mainly because of cultural differences in diet. Asians have a lower rate of osteoporosis than do Americans, and the Japanese are able to live with a much lower bone density than ours and still not sustain osteoporotic fractures. Much of this difference is most likely a result of a diet that's high in bone boosting soy foods. But a seeming contradiction exists, given that dairy intake is often *lower* in those countries that have a decreased risk of osteoporosis. We'll examine this paradox in chapters to come.

How Osteoporosis Causes Fractures

Fractures are by far the most serious complication of osteoporosis. The three most common types of fractures are spinal compression fractures; hip fractures; and wrist fractures. Because of their far-reaching implications in long-term health, it makes sense to understand how they work.

Spinal Compression Fractures

We've all seen the old lady in the shopping mall or at the produce stand who is so hunched over that she's nearly bent double. This disfiguring affliction is the outward sign of compression fractures in the spine and is caused by osteoporosis. As the condition we call "dowager's hump" worsens, the sufferer goes from being slightly stooped to being so bent over that she's forced to look downward all the time. In order to see where she's going, she has to hold her neck in a hyperextended position, causing further orthopedic maladies. Neck pain is a common complication, and there is usually an acceleration of arthritis in the bones of the neck. (See Figure 3-1.)

Because compression fractures are so common—by the age of eighty-five, most women will have at least one compression fracture in their spine—it's worth examining the mechanism of the spinal column.

The spine, of course, supports the body and bears its weight. There are twenty-four vertebrae in the spine—seven in the cervical (neck) area, twelve in the thoracic (chest) area, and five in the lumbar (lower back) area. There is also a sacrum and coccyx attached to the vertebral column. **Vertebral disks** are shock absorbing structures that separate the vertebrae. These can occasionally rupture and put pressure on the spinal nerves that lie nearby—a condition known as a **herniated disk,** or **slipped disk.**

The vertebrae are composed primarily of spongy bone, as opposed to harder, compact bone. Spongy bone is extremely active from a metabolic standpoint—that is, it goes through the process of breaking down and rebuilding more often than other types of bone, and as such is more vulnerable. The vertebrae are a primary site for the manifestations of osteoporosis, and we see this in the form of compression fractures.

Visualize a typical vertebra as a hatbox—it's soft on the inside and supported on its periphery by a rim of compact bone. If you sat down on one end of a hatbox, that end would be crunched down and the hatbox would assume a wedge shape. This is what

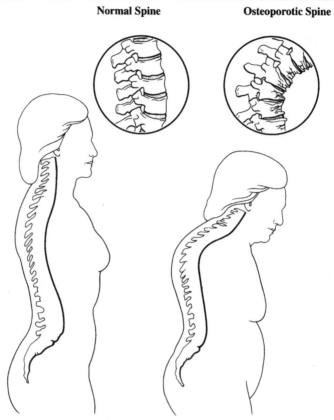

Figure 3-1. Normal and osteoporotic spines. *Reprinted with permission from the National Osteoporosis Foundation, Washington, D.C.*

happens in a compression fracture. The front of the vertebra, or the anterior surface, becomes shortened in relation to the rear, or posterior surface, as a result of the compression fracture.

Compression fractures carry with them an additional but remote risk of spinal cord damage—a condition that's extremely rare in osteoporosis-related compression fractures. It's also possible, and common, for younger people who don't have osteoporosis to develop compression fractures of the spine as a result of trauma (such as an automobile accident or a fall from a height). In these cases, it's more common for the hard back of the vertebrae, or posterior surface, to be driven into the spinal cord, causing significant nerve damage or even paralysis. Most osteoporotic compression fractures, on the other hand, result predominantly in a deformed vertebra and severe pain. (See Figure 3-2.)

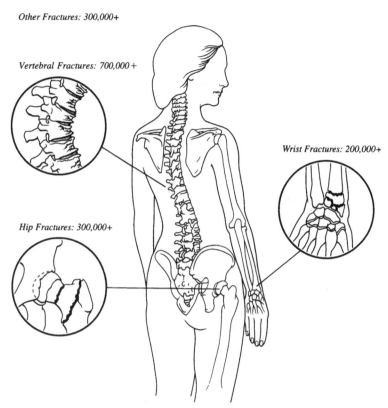

Other Fractures: 300,000+

Vertebral Fractures: 700,000+

Wrist Fractures: 200,000+

Hip Fractures: 300,000+

Figure 3-2. Bone fracture areas. Reprinted with permission from the National Osteoporosis Foundation, Washington, D.C.

Hip Fractures

It's a well-known fact that hip fractures are common in older people. A fifty-year-old woman has about a 20 percent chance of dealing with a hip fracture before she dies. Nearly one-third of women in their eighties will sustain a hip fracture.

The hips are made up of more hard bone (called cortical bone) than the vertebrae. This hard bone isn't as pliable or as flexible as vertebrae, and, is therefore more prone to breakage. Elderly people sometimes have an unsteady gait and are more prone to falls, often landing on one side and fracturing the relatively delicate hip bone. Generally, the bone is already significantly weakened by osteoporosis, and a relatively small trauma can cause a fracture. The weight of the body falling on an osteoporotic hip bone is more than enough to cause a break. (See Figure 3-2.)

Wrist Fractures

Wrist fractures related to osteoporosis are nearly as common as hip fractures—there are about a quarter of a million cases of each every year. Like the hips, the wrist has more cortical bone than the vertebrae. Also like the hips, the wrists are more likely to sustain fractures because of falls, common among older people with an unsteady gait. When we fall, we instinctively try to brace ourselves by putting out a hand. In normal circumstances, our wrist bones are sufficiently strong to absorb the impact. If those bones are weakened, as they are in osteoporosis, they can't withstand the weight of the fall and they fracture easily. This kind of break is commonly referred to as Colles fracture. (See Figure 3-2.)

Phases in the Development of Bone

In the first two chapters, we discussed the formation of bone throughout life. Now that we're specifically discussing osteoporosis, let's break that formation down into stages. Our bone mass changes in three primary phases during our lifetime, and by understanding each, we can see how osteoporosis may be prevented.

• *The first phrase in our bone development is the attainment of peak bone mass.* Our skeletal system develops rapidly during the growing years, and typically reaches its maximum size and density between ages twenty and thirty. Many factors have an effect on our peak bone mass, including gender, heredity, nutrition, and physical activity. The idea is to achieve the highest bone mass and denser bones in childhood and through early adulthood. After you achieve peak bone mass, the secret is knowing how to maintain it in order to avoid osteoporosis. We'll show you how to do this in the chapters to come.

• *The second phase in our skeletal life (starting about age thirty-five) consists of a gradual bone loss.* Osteoporosis is a degenerative disease. As we age, our bones thin, and the body doesn't repair them in an appropriate manner. Obviously, the less successful you've been at achieving a high peak bone mass early in life, the more significant your risks for bone disease are in your midthirties. The good news is, it's not too late. Preventive measures are now being embraced not only by alternative practitioners but also by the medical community. All those reports about the significance of vitamin D, estrogen, and other factors in the development of osteoporosis are finally being recognized.

• *The third phase of bone mass change generally occurs in postmenopausal women (around the age of fifty or so).* It's when bone density is at its lowest, and osteoporotic breaks are most apt to occur. This stage has traditionally been considered inevitable by physicians, but we'll look at ways to treat osteoporosis through diet, exercise, and lifestyle.

Primary and Secondary Osteoporosis

Osteoporosis is generally broken down into two types: primary and secondary. Simply speaking, **primary osteoporosis** is what most physicians consider a normal process of aging. It typically has its onset prior to menopause and gets worse after menopause. **Secondary osteoporosis** is typically associated with one of several different known causes. These include hormonal activity, prescription drugs, connective tissue disorders, and gastrointestinal disorders. Other causes include such well-known high-risk factors as smoking, prolonged immobilization, and lack of exercise.

Primary Osteoporosis

Primary osteoporosis generally starts somewhere between the ages of thirty and forty, and is marked by a slow, relentless bone loss. Women typically begin to experience significant bone loss following menopause, when the ovaries stop producing estrogen and progesterone and the resulting hormonal deficiency accelerates bone loss. Interestingly, estrogen and progesterone deficiency—and the consequent bone loss—are also common in female athletes who cease to menstruate, and in women who have had their ovaries removed at the same time they had a hysterectomy. Studies have shown significantly lower bone density in the vertebrae of serious female athletes. If you're one of these women, don't think you have to give up—just be aware that you may be at higher risk, and follow the suggestions in this book to keep your bones in shape.

Secondary Osteoporosis

A discussion of all the causes of secondary osteoporosis is beyond the scope of this book, but a few of the most significant and relevant factors should be examined. These are examined in greater detail in later chapters.

• **Calcium** A strategic nutrient in the prevention and treatment program of osteoporosis. Studies have shown that bone loss can be slowed by simply increasing calcium intake from 400 mg per day to 800 mg per day. The current Recommended Daily Allowance (RDA) for calcium is 1200 mg a day for both men and women, and 1500 mg a day for postmenopausal women who are not being treated for osteoporosis. Women who are taking estrogen replacement therapy may get by with an intake of 1000 mg daily.

Even though calcium is only one of the many minerals necessary for healthy bones, it's an important one. And the fact of the matter is, most women don't get enough calcium. In one study, postmenopausal women, who require 1500 mg of calcium daily, had an intake of only about 500 mg daily. Many or most women—and men—on a so-called normal diet are calcium-deficient. And eating enough calcium doesn't necessarily mean *absorbing* enough calcium: various factors, including caffeine and sugar, can make calcium less available to the body.

• **Smoking** If you don't already have enough reasons to shun smoking, add osteoporosis to the list. As we've seen, estrogen helps prevent osteoporosis by inhibiting the action of osteoclasts, the cells that break down bone. Smoking, on the other hand, is known to *inactivate* estrogen and create a relative estrogen deficiency. Smokers hit menopause an average of almost two years before nonsmokers. In addition, smokers are typically sedentary and less likely to pursue exercise as an essential life activity, further accelerating the development of osteoporosis.

• **Caffeine** America's love affair with coffee may prove to be a fatal attraction after all: caffeine has a direct effect on the body's mineral content by causing the body to excrete calcium and other minerals. At high levels, caffeine can lower blood calcium and magnesium enough to stimulate bone breakdown, and other minerals are lost as well. A definite association has been demonstrated between increased caffeine intake and a higher incidence of hip fractures in women. One or two cups a day is probably safe, but any more than that could be detrimental.

• **Alcohol** The issue of alcohol consumption has become a hot topic as a result of recent studies definitively linking moderate alcohol consumption to a lower incidence of death from heart disease and stroke. The term "moderate" has typically been defined as two drinks per day. What's not mentioned in these studies is the fact that alcohol has a definite, deleterious role in hastening the development of osteoporosis.

People who use alcohol excessively tend to be malnourished and are likely to have an inadequate intake of bone-essential minerals. Additionally, excessive alcohol consumption can lead to decreased vitamin D metabolism because of liver damage. It has also been postulated that alcohol directly damages the bone forming cells, thereby hampering the formation of bone. Another point to consider: alcohol leads to impaired judgment and mobility, so the risk of sustaining a bone breaking fall is much higher. If you're having a glass of wine a few times a week, you probably don't need to worry. But if you're a daily drinker, you might want to consider curbing your habit.

The Causes of Secondary Osteoporosis

A number of factors—some within our control, some not—can affect our risk of developing osteoporosis. Certain substances, medications, and diseases have the side effect of increasing the risk of osteoporosis. If you've been diagnosed with any of the diseases listed here, or you're taking any of the medications listed, talk to your physician about beginning complementary therapies to enhance your bone health.

Factors That Increase the Risk of Osteoporosis

Medical Conditions

- Acromegaly
- Cushing's syndrome
- Diabetes mellitus
- Ehrlers-Danlos syndrome
- Gasterectomy
- Hepatobilliary disease and cirrhosis
- Homocysternuria
- Hyperthyroidism
- Hypogonadism
- Hypothyroidism
- Intestinal by-pass surgery
- Malabsorption
- Marfan's syndrome
- Menkes' syndrome
- Osteogenesis imperfecta
- Scurvy

Drugs

- Alcohol
- Aluminum-containing antacids
- Anticonvulsants
- Caffeine
- Corticosteroids
- GNRH agonist
- Heparin
- Isoniazid
- Lasix
- Lithium
- Methotrexate
- Progesterone
- Thyroid hormone

Other Risk Factors

- Dietary mineral deficiencies
- Genetic predisposition
- Immobilization
- Lack of exercise
- Smoking

Estrogen, Progesterone, and Osteoporosis

We've already reviewed some of the associations between estrogen deficiency and osteoporosis. Now let's take a closer look at this crucial hormone. Estrogen is the female hormone which is required for the development of specifically female characteristics. It's responsible for the normal maturation of the vagina and uterus, and the development of what are called secondary female sexual characteristics, including breasts and the distribution of body fat that we associate with the female shape.

Various metabolic effects, like the maintenance of normal skin texture and the integrity of blood vessels, are dependent on estrogen. Estrogen also lowers LDL (the "bad" cholesterol) levels and raises HDL (the "good" cholesterol) levels, resulting in a lower incidence of death from heart disease.

Estrogen also plays a vital role in the development and treatment of osteoporosis. Numerous medical studies dating back almost sixty years document the vital role of estrogen deficiency in the development of osteoporosis. There are also a number of theories about how estrogen prevents osteoporosis, some of which we've discussed in previous chapters. To review:

- Estrogens are known to decrease the rate of bone breakdown.
- Estrogens block the effect of certain other hormones—particularly parathyroid hormone (PTH)—that break down bones.
- Estrogen binds to receptors on the surface of osteoclasts cells, preventing them from functioning in a normal fashion.

When women go through menopause, their ovaries stop producing estrogen. But levels of estrogen begin to drop many years before menopause. That drop, which starts in the midthirties, is a significant factor in the development of osteoporosis. In other words, it's not prudent to wait until menopause to start treating osteoporosis. Prevention must start far in advance—in fact, years in advance—of that point.

- **Progesterone** Taken either with or instead of estrogen, progesterone is beginning to be recognized and used to treat osteoporosis. It's a hormone produced by the ovaries that stimulates the action of osteoblasts, which build bone, and also helps decrease the withdrawal of calcium from bones. There's a growing belief that progesterone deficiency is associated with osteoporosis, and several studies have linked the two. Additionally, supplementation with progesterone has been found to correct bone loss. While initial reports of progesterone treatment are promising, more research is needed.

Other Crucial Hormones

Hormones are substances produced in the body by endocrine glands. They regulate many important bodily functions on a cellular level by acting as chemical messengers. Hormones work by interacting with receptors on the surface of many different cells, and they also have the ability to operate inside cells. Hormonal or endocrine disorders typically result from either an excess or a deficiency of the effects produced by the hormones. After they accomplish their goal of delivering messages to cells, hormones typically undergo a process of deactivation or transform into other hormones.

A number of endocrine glands can affect bones and therefore have a direct impact on the development of osteoporosis. The glands that primarily affect bones, and osteoporosis, include the thyroid, pituitary, and parathyroid.

The thyroid gland is in the front of the neck—it's the one your doctor palpates during your annual exam. The pituitary gland in the brain works in conjunction with the thyroid, secreting a substance called thyroid stimulating hormone (TSH) that helps the thyroid gland make hormones. The two hormones we're interested in are thyroxin and calcitonin.

Thyroxin is crucial not only to bone health, but also to the metabolism of all cells. If the body produces too much thyroxin, a condition results known as hyperthyroidism. If the body doesn't produce enough thyroxin, another kind of condition results, known as **hypothyroidism,** which is typically treated with a synthetic thyroid hormone. In either case, the net result is the same: too much thyroxin can lead to decreased bone mineral content and osteoporosis. If you've been diagnosed with hypothyroidism and are taking thyroid hormone, it's critical that your doctors routinely check your overall condition.

Calcitonin, the other hormone secreted by the thyroid, works by keeping osteoclasts from breaking down bone. The amount of calcitonin the body produces is directly controlled by the amount of calcium in the blood. Too much calcium in the blood, and calcitonin secretion is increased; too little, and calcitonin production is shut off. Calcitonin also affects the kidneys, increasing the excretion of calcium when calcium levels are too high.

The parathyroid glands, located in the neck on the back of the thyroid gland, produce a hormone called parathyroid hormone (PTH), which we discussed in earlier chapters. Remember that PTH works closely in conjunction with the hormone calcitonin, produced by the thyroid gland. Typically PTH removes calcium from the bones in response to a low calcium level in the blood. Calcitonin, on the other hand, has the ability to add calcium to the bones if blood calcium levels are too high. To maintain this delicate balance, there must be enough calcium in one's diet.

The hormone PTH also stimulates the synthesis of vitamin D, which acts as a hormone inside the body. The mechanism of action is intricate and complex. Here's a quick review of how it works:

1. Vitamin D is synthesized in the skin with the help of sunlight or from dietary sources, and is in a form called cholecalciferol (vitamin D_3).
2. For vitamin D to become fully active and help us absorb calcium, it has to be transformed into a different form. Two more chemi-

cal reactions take place: first in the liver and second in the kidneys.
3. The result is the most active form of vitamin D (1,25-dihydroxy-cholecalciferol, for you science buffs), which is what we really need for bone health.
4. The main action of this active form of vitamin D is to accelerate calcium and phosphate absorption from the intestine, thus increasing the amount of calcium we have circulating in our blood and decreasing the likelihood that calcium will be stolen from the bones.

Diseases Related to Bone Density

As we've seen, the skeletal system is related to all systems of the body. Consequently, a number of common, and not so common, diseases can affect bone density and thus, osteoporosis. Following are some diseases and disorders that may have an impact on bone health.

• **Diabetes** A potentially fatal disease that stems from a deficiency of insulin secretion in the body and it manifests in two types. The first, called Type I, or insulin-dependent diabetes, is treated with regular doses of extra insulin. The second, Type II, or noninsulin-dependent diabetes, doesn't usually require insulin treatments. For reasons not yet known, people with insulin-dependent diabetes are more likely to have osteoporosis and osteoporotic fractures than those with noninsulin-dependent diabetes and much less frequently suffer from osteoporosis. Interestingly, studies have shown that women with noninsulin dependent diabetes actually have *higher* bone mineral densities than those with no disease.

• **Cushing's disease** A condition in which cortisone is over-produced by the adrenal glands. Cortisone is a type of steroid, and steroids are strongly associated with osteoporosis. We'll go into more detail about this later in the chapter. In the meantime, suffice it to say that any condition that causes an increase in cortisone in the body is definitely linked to osteoporosis.

• **Hypogonadism** A condition in which there is a decrease in the amount of sex hormones. In men, this results in a decrease in testosterone, the male hormone, a condition that's been associated with osteoporosis. In women, this results in chronic estrogen deficiency, and osteoporosis is common since estrogen loss is one of the causes of bone loss.

• **Connective tissue disorders** Also called autoimmune disorders. These disorders result in chronic, widespread inflammation of connective tissues in the body and frequently in immune system changes. Two examples of connective tissue disorders are lupus and rheumatoid arthritis. Because of their effect on the immune system, osteoporosis is common in people with connective tissue disorders.

• **Gastrectomy** The medical term for surgery to remove all or part of the stomach, generally because of trauma, cancer, or other disease. One of the most significant side effects of gastrectomy is the development of osteoporosis. The absorption of calcium and vitamin D is compromised, and the production of PTH is increased, leading to calcium loss from the bones.

• **Intestinal bypass surgery** This procedure, in which a section of the small intestine is sectioned off and reconnected, became a briefly popular solution for massive obesity. The small intestine is responsible for the proper absorption of nutrients, so when portions of it are unavailable, the absorption of calcium and vitamin D is compromised. There are a few cases in which intestinal bypass surgery is necessary, as in extreme trauma, but unless it's a life threatening circumstance, the procedure is generally ill advised.

• **Malabsorption** A broad term that encompasses many disease processes in which nutrients aren't absorbed because of a malfunction in the digestive processes. The intestinal tract may be damaged by Crohn's disease or sprue. Because the absorption of calcium and other nutrients is compromised, the end result can be osteoporosis.

• **Genetic conditions** A variety of genetic diseases that affect the synthesis of bone can lead to osteoporosis. In these conditions, there is basically a defect in the formation of the bone matrix itself. Some of the diseases in this category include osteogenesis imperfecta, Ehrlers-Danlos syndrome, homocystinuria, Menkes' syndrome, and Marfan's syndrome.

Drugs That May Cause Osteoporosis

While drugs do have their place in modern medicine, many common medications taken by millions of people on a regular basis have all kinds of nasty side effects—including osteoporosis. Some of these drugs are necessary in emergency situations, and others can alleviate excruciating pain; steroids and corticosteroids, for example, can save the life of a shock victim and make life bearable for arthritis sufferers. But unless they're truly necessary for survival, you're probably better off without them.

Some physicians may take the easy way out and prescribe commonly used drugs. They may not know about or believe in complementary therapies. Seek out a physician who's versed in complementary therapies, or at least get a second opinion from another doctor.

It all becomes a matter of weighing the side effects against the benefits, a decision that can only be made by you and your health care practitioner. And while you're weighing, remember that there are natural substitutes for many or most of the medications listed below. Following are some of the most commonly prescribed drugs that cause osteoporosis:

• **Corticosteroids** Generally used to treat inflammatory disorders like rheumatoid arthritis, corticosteroids come in many forms. Some of the more common ones are cortisone, prednisone, prednisolone, and dexamethasone. All of them have been definitely linked with osteoporosis.

Steroids are bad for bones for several different reasons. They inhibit calcium absorption and increase the loss of calcium. They decrease the body's ability to synthesis collagen, part of the protein matrix needed to produce bone. They're also known to lower estrogen levels, increasing the likelihood of osteoporosis. And studies have shown that steroids can inhibit the action of osteoblasts, the cells that form bone.

Unfortunately, it usually doesn't take a tremendous amount of steroid medication to create significant side effects. Some studies have shown that even steroid-containing inhalers for allergies can harm bone health. Which is not to imply that steroids should be banned from medical use altogether. Steroids can be lifesavers in such situations as shock, and they offer substantial relief for those who suffer from severe arthritis and collagen disorders. They also may be the only answer for some disorders, like lupus. It's a trade-off and a difficult decision, but some people may have to risk the side effects of osteoporosis to deal with unbearably painful or life threatening diseases.

• **GNRH agonists** GNRH stands for the gonadotropin-releasing hormones that are produced in the pituitary gland. GNRH agonists, the synthetic forms of these hormones, are used to treat endometriosis—a painful thickening of the walls of the endometrium. They work by creating temporary ovarian failure, which causes estrogen levels to fall and can lead to osteoporosis. On the positive side, they're not generally used on a long-term basis, and the decrease in bone density that results from their use has been shown to be reversible.

• **Methotrexate** A drug that has become popular for treating cancer, but people who take methotrexate for a long period of time generally develop osteoporosis. While methotrexate, a chemotherapy agent, is effective in treating cancer, it can cause osteoporosis by interfering with the function of the osteoblasts that form bone and by stimulating bone breakdown.

• **Lithium** A drug commonly used to treat manic-depressive disorder, a psychiatric illness that's prevalent in the United States. Lithium has a great success rate in treating manic depression, but it can also increase the production of PTH and thus lead to osteoporosis.

• **Dilantin** An anticonvulsant used to treat seizure disorders like epilepsy. While extremely effective in preventing seizures, Dilantin also increases PTH production, decreases the production of vitamin D, and interferes with calcium absorption. The net effect is osteoporosis.

• **Isoniazid** An antibiotic used to treat tuberculosis, a highly contagious respiratory condition that's on the rise in the United States. One of its unfortunate side effects is an increased loss of calcium and a greater risk of osteoporosis.

What It All Means

As you read through this chapter, you probably found that some of the risk factors for osteoporosis apply to you—maybe you just drink too much coffee, or maybe you're on Dilantin to treat epilepsy. Some of these risk factors can be changed, some cannot. While we can't alter our genetic makeup, we *can* drink less coffee and alcohol, and we can stop smoking. Lifestyle habits, both good and bad, are learned behaviors. It's simply a matter of applying knowledge and discipline to eliminate the risk factors we can control and thus reduce the overall risk of osteoporosis.

4

DIAGNOSING OSTEOPOROSIS

In the previous chapters, we've spoken of treatments for osteoporosis—both traditional and complementary. But no matter how you choose to treat any disease, including osteoporosis, you won't get far without a complete and accurate diagnosis. Even though this book is aimed at nontraditional treatments, let's not kid ourselves: in terms of diagnosing illness, nothing beats Western medicine. The technology is unsurpassed, as are the skills of most diagnostic physicians. The key is to use the best of both worlds, and to choose a doctor carefully.

A physician has the most privileged listening post a human can have. In the doctor-patient relationship we are, after all, talking about matters of life and death. Your doctor should listen to, and really hear, your issues and concerns about medication, treatment methods, and so forth. If you're not being heard, speak up and voice your concerns. If you're not comfortable doing that, it's time to get a new physician. If your doctor is not open to complementary medicine, he or she may be doing you more harm than good. And remember your job as a patient: you need to be completely open and honest, about everything from how much coffee you drink to your level of exercise. You must also voice your concerns or fears about any medications you may be taking or are about to take.

In a perfect world, doctors would be able to take the time to educate their patients about osteoporosis and the treatments available. But doctors are busy people, and because of the way our modern medical system is set up, they can't devote as much time and care as you may need. So it's up to you to take control and to become as educated as possible on your own. Let's look at some of the questions your doctor should be asking, the procedures that mark an effective diagnosis and treatment, and the role you can take in helping to devise your course of natural and complementary treatment.

Talking to Your Doctor

Any form of medical treatment must start with a comprehensive history and physical examination. Here's where the patient's role becomes critical, and this first step is the area in which the doctor-patient relationship begins to unfold.

Defining the Pain

Unless we're going in for a routine physical or annual exam, most of us see a doctor because of pain. Osteoporosis usually shows up first as back pain, generally between the lower borders of the shoulder blades. But pain is relative, and many factors are involved. When you're describing pain or discomfort, be aware of your body and focus in on the specifics. Let's assume you're seeing a doctor because of back pain. Think about the following questions so you can help your doctor make the most comprehensive diagnosis:

- **Location of the pain** Try to pinpoint as best you can where the pain is centered. Rather than saying, "My back hurts," be more specific. Is it the lower couple of inches of your spine? Is it in the center or more toward the edges?
- **Nature of the pain** What kind of pain do you feel in your back? Try to define it: stabbing, throbbing, cramping, dull, sharp, and so forth.
- **Timing of the pain** Does your back hurt all the time, or is the pain intermittent? If so, how often does it hurt, and for how long? Does it wake you up at night?
- **Radiation of the pain** If your back hurts, does the pain stay in one location, or does it tend to move around? If so, when and in what direction?
- **Severity of the pain** Using a scale of one to ten is helpful in determining the relative severity of any kind of pain.
- **Factors that make the pain worse** Does your back hurt more when you're standing or lying down? Does movement increase or decrease the pain? What about heat or cold?

So, using this example: instead of saying, "My back hurts," you'd say, "My lower back hurts, right on the spine. It's a dull, throbbing pain that comes and goes about every two hours, and it tends to move downward. It's usually about a seven on a scale of one to ten."

Using a heating pad makes it feel better, but it hurts more when I'm lying on my back." By being as specific as possible, you can help your doctor make the most accurate diagnosis.

Talking About Your History

Your past medical history is critical and should include a thorough listing of any diseases you've been treated for, any medications you're taking now, and medications you've taken in the past. As we've seen, a number of diseases and medications are related to osteoporosis. Social history is just as important. Tell your doctor, honestly, how much and how often you drink alcohol, whether you smoke and if so how much, and what your caffeine intake is like. These are just a few of the factors that play a critical role in the development of osteoporosis.

Having a Physical Exam

During the poking and prodding portion of the exam, your doctor should determine the range of motion of your arms, check for muscle spasms by palpating the tender area, and press on bone to feel the spine. Ideally, you should have a comprehensive exam every year, along with a blood chemistry profile (BCP).

Making the Diagnosis

After taking a complete history and doing a physical examination, the doctor's next step will be taking an X ray to find out if you have any fractures. The term *bone density* refers to the amount of bone mineral within a cubic centimeter of bone. The density of the bone is responsible for the strength of the bone and the resistance to fracture.

Diagnosing Fractures

Plain X rays are commonly used to study the skeletal structure, but they're not effective in diagnosing osteoporosis. In the case of osteoporosis, bones look washed out and less opaque on a plain X ray. (See Figures 4-1 and 4-2 for a comparison of normal and osteoporotic spine X rays.) But osteoporosis doesn't show up on an X ray until a third or more of the bone mass is lost—a considerable decrease. In other words, by the time osteoporosis shows up on an X ray, substantial bone loss has already occurred. X rays are still used to diagnose fractures related to osteoporosis, but the diagnosis of osteoporosis itself is made by using variations on the plain X ray. We'll talk about those in detail below.

Fractures of the Vertebrae

When the vertebrae are X-rayed, signs of osteoporosis show up in a number of different ways. Hard bone forms the outside of the vertebra. Spongy bone makes up the inside of the vertebra and is more susceptible to osteoporosis. When the spongy bone on the inside of the vertebra starts to disappear, the result is a "picture frame appearance": the outline of the vertebra appears, but the inside is barely visible.

Another sign of osteoporosis shows up in the disks. The vertebrae in the back are separated by disks made of cartilage that act as shock absorbers. When the bone of the vertebra becomes softer, as it does in osteoporosis, the disk may herniate or move into the vertebra itself. In this case, the bottom and top of the vertebra have a curved appearance.

One of the most common presentations of osteoporosis in the spinal area is a compression fracture of the vertebra. In this case, when the vertebra is seen from the side, the front surface is lower in height than the back surface, and the vertebra has what is known as **anterior wedging**. (See Figures 4-3 and 4-4.) Fractures of the back surface of the vertebrae are uncommon in osteoporosis. If your doctor finds fractures in this area, he or she will likely look for cancer, rather than osteoporosis, in the bone.

Fractures of the Wrist and Hip

The hip and wrist are the other sites typically involved in osteoporosis. Osteoporosis of the hip or wrist, however, is very difficult to diagnose on a plain X ray because there is much more cortical bone in these areas than in the vertebrae. Since osteoporosis affects cortical bone much less than it affects a spongy bone, it doesn't readily reveal itself on X rays of the hip and wrist until a fracture appears.

Measuring Bone Density

Because X rays can detect osteoporosis only in relatively advanced stages, the only reliable way to diagnose osteoporosis is by directly measuring bone density. The technology that enables doctors to measure bone density has evolved rapidly since its inception more than thirty years ago and is extraordinarily accurate. In fact,

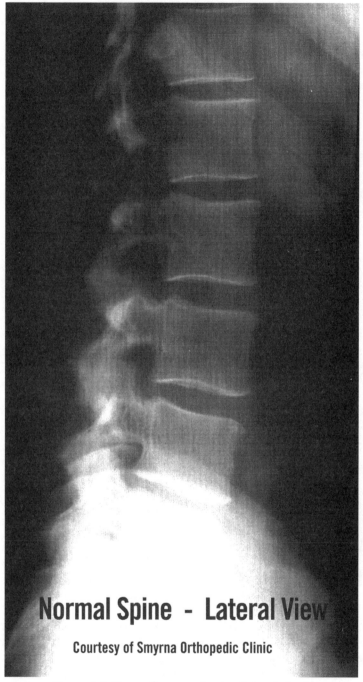

Figure 4-1. X ray of a normal spine (lateral view).

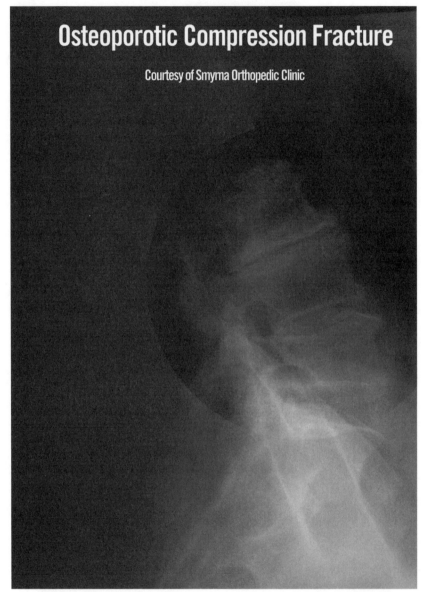

Figure 4-2. Osteoporotic compression fracture.

researchers have found that bone mass assessment was effective in detecting early signs of osteoporosis, thereby identifying people who were at greater risk of having a fracture.

Right now, there are several distinct methods to determine bone mineral density. One invasive but extremely accurate diagnostic

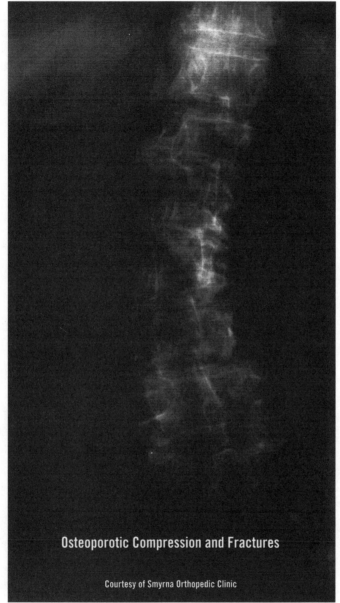

Osteoporotic Compression and Fractures

Courtesy of Smyrna Orthopedic Clinic

Figure 4-3. Osteoporotic compression and fractures.

technique involves taking a bone biopsy (a thin slice of bone), a nearly definitive method of identifying osteoporotic bone (See Figure 4-5.) Other procedures are less invasive and more commonly

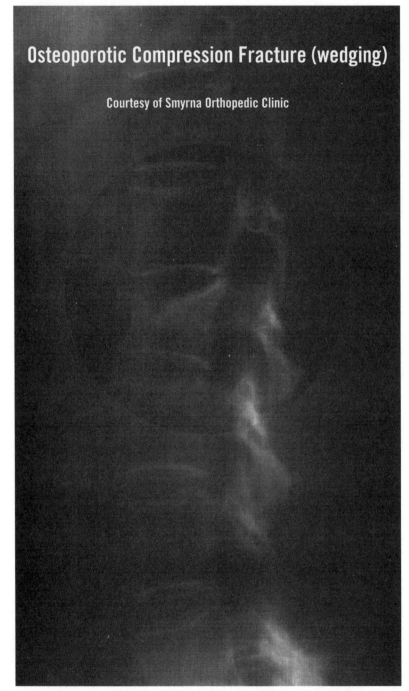

Figure 4-4. Osteoporotic compression fracture (wedging).

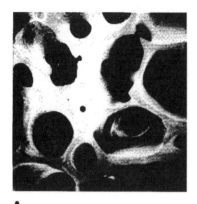 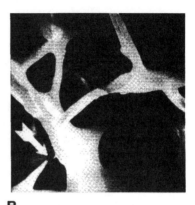

A   **B**

Micrographs of biopsy specimens of normal and osteoporotic bone. PANEL A is from a 75-year-old normal woman. PANEL B is from a 47-year-old woman who had multiple vertebral compression fractures.

Figure 4-5. Micrographs of biopsy specimens of normal and osteoporotic bone.

used. Of these, some are more accurate than others, and none of them are able to determine the cause of the bone loss itself. They all, however, help doctors formulate an effective treatment protocol based on their results.

The four primary methods using X rays are radiographic absorptiometry (RA), single energy X ray absorptiometry (SXA), duel energy absorptiometry (DXA), and quantitative computed tomography (QCT). In addition, ultrasound densitometry may provide some measure of bone density. We're going to get into some fairly technical information, so bear with us. It will help you understand which diagnostic treatment your doctor is using, and give you tools for taking part in your diagnosis.

• **Radiographic absorptiometry (RA)** This is the simplest technique, since it can be performed in a doctor's office with a regular X-ray machine. RAs can only be used to X-ray the hand, and are used primarily to determine the relative overall health of bone. An X ray is taken of the hand next to a piece of aluminum. After the film is developed, it is interpreted with the aluminum serving as a reference for density. A special scanner calculates the density of the bones in the fingers. This technique allows doctors to determine bone density precisely, using standard X-ray equipment, long before 30 percent of the bone is gone.

• **Single-energy X-ray absorptiometry (SXA)** This technique is commonly used, but can only measure those bones near the surface that aren't surrounded by large amounts of soft tissue, like fat or muscle. For this reason, it has profound limitations and is usually used only to diagnose bone density of the wrist and the heel. The hip and spine can't be effectively examined with SXA—a significant drawback because osteoporosis typically shows up in the spine. Additionally, the mortality rate from hip fractures far exceeds the complications associated with osteoporotic fractures of the spine or wrist. For this reason, many doctors don't opt for SXA. In general, it can be used as an indicator of relative bone health.

Since soft tissue can interfere with the ability to measure bone density effectively and see bones on an X-ray, SXAs use different methods to make bones more visible. In the SXA technique, the heel or wrist is immersed in a bath of water to simulate uniform soft tissue thickness. A single energy X-ray beam, as opposed to a dual beam, is then used to image the skeletal site and bone density is determined.

• **Dual-energy X-ray absorptiometry (DXA or DEXA)** This is by far the most reliable diagnostic tool for osteoporosis. DXA was developed in the 1980s and its widespread use began in 1988. This state-of-the-art technique is considered the best method to check bone density in all areas of the body, even in those areas covered heavily by soft tissue—a distinct advantage over the SXA technique.

In DXA, two X-ray beams are used, and the procedure is able to subtract the soft tissue absorption and calculate accurate bone mineral densities in deep sites. This fact enables doctors to image both the spine and the hip—a critically important factor, since fractures in the spine and hip are the most serious and disabling. DXA can determine if a person's bone mass is typical for his or her age and whether he or she has a significant risk of fractures.

Another advantage is that the DXA scan is extremely precise and can detect subtle changes in bone density that may occur from year to year. For this reason, it may be wise for women to get a baseline DXA scan that can then serve as a reference point to determine loss of bone density as they grow older. Additionally, DXAs allow the physician to determine whether the therapies or treatments being used are working, based on initial baselines.

• **Quantitative computed tomography (QCT)** QCT uses the same technology as computed tomography, or CAT scan. QCTs provide highly accurate measurements of bone density and are generally used for the spine. The primary advantage of QCTs is that they can measure the center of the bone, which is affected first and most severely. The primary disadvantage is the higher exposure to radiation and the expense.

Most radiologists and endocrinologists feel that QCT is able to provide an accurate measurement of spongy bone density, even in the center of the vertebra itself. QCT is the only bone mineral density measurement that provides true three-dimensional measurements. Since osteoporosis involves predominantly spongy bone, QCT can be a helpful diagnostic tool.

• **Ultrasound densitometry** This technique is similar to the ultrasound technique. which has wide applications in obstetrics, abdominal surgery, and vascular studies. Ultrasound densitometry has become popular in some circles for determining bone density. Some studies indicate that ultrasound can accurately predict fracture risk, including the possibility of hip fracture and vertebral fractures. This could be extremely helpful, considering the serious ramifications of both hip and vertebral fractures. But most doctors feel that ultrasound techniques aren't sufficiently accurate in diagnosing osteoporosis.

PRIMARY METHODS TO MEASURE BONE DENSITY

Method	Advantages	Disadvantages
Radiographic absorptiometry (RA)	Simplest technique to determine overall bone health.	Limited to X rays of the hand.
Single-energy X-ray absorptiometry (SXA)	Commonly used to indicate relative bone health.	Can only measure bones near the surface. Cannot measure hip or spine.
Dual-energy X-ray absorptiometry	Most reliable method to check bone density in all areas of the body.	

(DXA, DEXA)	Extremely precise; can determine subtle changes in bone density.	
Quantitative computed tomography	Highly accurate. Can measure the center of the bone, which is usually affected first in osteoporosis.	High exposure to radiation. Expensive.
Ultrasound densitometry	Can help predict fracture risk.	Not very accurate in diagnosing osteoporosis

The tests listed above are the doctor's primary tools for diagnosing osteoporosis. Some are more accurate than others, but all can provide good diagnostic tools. Your doctor will tell you, based on your personal condition and situation, which test or combination of tests, is best for you.

How DXAs Work

The DXA diagnostic procedure works by computing what's known as a **T-score** and a **Z-score**. The T-score compares your bone density with that of an average thirty-year-old. The Z-score compares your bone density with that of other people your own age and sex. The comparison of the two figures is a fairly accurate determination of bone-loss percentage, assuming that you had a normal bone density at the age of thirty.

You might have a bone mineral density similar to people your own age, and you may still have osteoporosis and an increased risk of fractures because of other factors. For this reason, only the T-score is used to determine if you have osteoporosis and increased risk of fracture. If both numbers reveal that more bone is being lost than would normally be expected, your doctor will probably order a complete evaluation.

DXA scans are advisable for women entering menopause to establish a baseline and determine how much bone they're losing over subsequent years. Additionally, DXA scans are helpful for people who have taken steroids for a prolonged period of time. In either case, if the DXA scan shows that bone density is declining too rapidly, alternative treatment plans can be entertained.

What It All Means

Osteoporosis is a multifaceted disease with several manifestations and many treatment methods. The cornerstone of any good treatment protocol, however, is an accurate diagnosis. In most cases, you'll probably rely on traditional medical approaches for diagnosing osteoporosis; they're the most advanced and accurate methods available. But that doesn't mean you have to accept traditional treatment. In the next chapter, we'll talk about how osteoporosis has been treated in the past, the shortcomings of traditional treatments and the dangers of drugs used for osteoporosis. The chapters after that will talk about new, natural approaches that offer a safe and effective treatment for osteoporosis.

5

TRADITIONAL TREATMENTS FOR OSTEOPOROSIS

We've painted a pretty grim picture of osteoporosis so far, and for good reason. It's a deadly disease with painful and far-reaching consequences. But don't give up hope—there are ways to prevent and treat osteoporosis. And it's never too late to reverse the effects of osteoporosis with safe and natural treatments. If you already have osteoporosis, or you're in a high-risk group, it's up to you to get busy and take charge of your life.

In this chapter we'll be talking about *traditional* treatments for osteoporosis, ranging from the basic lifestyle changes your doctor will probably recommend to prescription medications. As you read this, bear in mind that we're not necessarily endorsing these measures. Instead, we're presenting them so that you can compare them to the new approach, based on natural supplements, that we'll be exploring later. And if you're *currently* being treated within the parameters of the traditional medical community, it's important that you know as much as you can about what you're getting.

After you've been diagnosed with osteoporosis, it's up to you to work with your doctor to devise a treatment plan. You may choose to go with a nutritionally oriented physician for a more comprehensive complementary approach. Or your current doctor may be open to exploring various natural solutions. In the second half of this book, we'll show you how you can use diet, exercise, and a remarkable new nutritional supplement to build healthy bone and stop the progression of osteoporosis.

Diet and Nutritional Supplements

Even in the traditional medical community, the role of diet and nutrition in osteoporosis is widely recognized. Unfortunately, the primary focus has usually been on calcium and vitamin D. Yes, they're important factors, but as we'll see, a multitude of other vitamins, minerals, and nutrients are equally necessary for good bone health. But first, let's take a look at the more traditional medical approach to dietary supplements as a way of preventing and treating osteoporosis.

Calcium

The general medical community stresses ample calcium as the cornerstone to building stronger bones to prevent osteoporosis later in life. It's true that most people who suffer from osteoporosis have a decreased intake of calcium, and we Americans in general have a less-than-ideal intake of calcium. Recent studies show that up to two-thirds of the population is calcium deficient. The average calcium intake of a sixty-five-year-old woman is 550 mg a day— significantly lower than the recommended daily allowance of 1500 mg a day. But calcium isn't the only bone mineral:

The emphasis on calcium intake is often short-sighted, since many other minerals and nutrients are also important for the health of bone tissue and the prevention and treatment of osteoporosis.

Your doctor will probably suggest that you up your intake of milk and other dairy products. But a milk mustache isn't the only dietary answer to your calcium needs. Other foods can provide as much calcium as dairy—greens, for example, have about the same amount of calcium as milk—in a form that's more easily absorbed by your body. We'll talk about lots of other ways to add calcium to your diet in Chapter 6.

Your doctor may also recommend calcium supplements, especially if you're in a high-risk group for osteoporosis. Again, while calcium *is* important for healthy bones, it's only one of a broad spectrum of nutrients needed. In Chapter 7, we'll talk about all the nutrients needed for healthy bones. Meanwhile, be aware that there are risks associated with taking too much calcium, especially since it can interfere with the body's ability to use other important nutrients.

- Too much calcium will block the uptake of manganese and interfere with the absorption of magnesium, which is also important for bone health.
- Excessive calcium intake has been associated with decreased iron absorption, with the possible side effect of anemia.

- Too much calcium will interfere with the absorption of zinc—important for both bone and immune system health.
- Calcium in very high doses may interfere with the synthesis of vitamin K, which is not only important for appropriate blood clotting, but also plays a key role in bone health.
- Extremely high doses of calcium (about 5 grams a day) can cause kidney disorders in susceptible people. If you have a history of kidney stones, make sure your doctor knows this before you start a regimen of calcium supplements.

How Much Calcium Is Enough?

Calcium needs vary according to age and certain risk factors. The National Institutes of Health recommends the following total calcium intakes, in all forms—dietary and supplemental.

- Children one to five years old: 800 mg a day
- Children six to ten years old: 800 mg to 1200 mg a day
- Adolescents: 1200 to 1500 mg a day
- Adults between the ages of twenty-five and fifty: 1000 mg a day
- Pregnant or lactating women: 1500 mg a day
- Women over fifty: 1500 mg a day

Vitamin D

In addition to calcium, your doctor will probably stress an adequate intake of vitamin D, which plays a major role in regulating how the body metabolizes calcium and phosphorus. For instance, without vitamin D, the body can't absorb calcium effectively—children who don't get enough vitamin D end up with soft, weak bones and teeth. And if vitamin D is lacking, the pituitary glands are stimulated to produce more PTH, which in turn stimulates bone breakdown.

But before you start popping pills, remember that vitamin D deficiency is rare. Because vitamin D is so readily available—we synthesize it in our skin from exposure to the sun—it's hard to be deprived of this important nutrient for very long. And a little sunshine goes a long way. Most people only need about fifteen minutes of sunshine three or four times a week to ensure that there's an adequate amount of vitamin D in their bodies.

Only in elderly people is vitamin D deficiency common—

because of a number of factors including limited exposure to the sun, compromised digestion, and decreased kidney and liver function. If you're in this high-risk group, your doctor may recommend a combination of calcium and vitamin D supplements as a baseline treatment for osteoporosis. A regimen of 400 IU to 800 IU of vitamin D per day has been shown to significantly reduce the rate of bone loss.

Dairy products, fish and fish liver oils, dandelion greens, liver, and sweet potatoes are all excellent sources of vitamin D. The recommended dosage for adults is 400 IU and for people over the age of sixty-five, up to 800 IU. If you're taking vitamin D supplements on your own, pay close attention to the dosages. Excessive vitamin D intake can be toxic, and you should not exceed the recommended dosage.

Other Vitamins and Minerals

As well-fed as we Americans appear to be, most of us don't eat a healthy, balanced diet. As a nation, we eat too much processed and packaged foods and not enough whole foods—fresh fruits and vegetables, grains, beans, and nuts. Take a full-spectrum multivitamin/mineral preparation to be on the safe side. And if you're at increased risk for osteoporosis, pay attention to the vitamins and minerals that have specific effects on bone above and beyond calcium. Several minerals play integral roles in building healthy bone, but their importance is generally downplayed in the face of all the attention devoted to calcium. Make sure your multivitamin contains the following bone-friendly minerals and trace nutrients:

- **Vitamin K** A well-known factor in blood clotting, this vitamin is also required by osteoblasts—the bone builders—to produce the proteins found in bone.
- **Vitamin C** This vitamin is essential for the production of collagen, part of the protein matrix that forms bone and helps give bone its elasticity.
- **Copper, manganese, boron, silicon, magnesium, and zinc** All these minerals are important for bone health, and a deficiency in any of them can lead to poor bone health.

Exercise and Other Physical Activity

In earlier chapters, we reviewed the role of strain on bones and the skeletal system. (When you put stress on your bones, they respond by getting stronger.) Putting stress on the skeletal system increases bone density and lowers the risk of osteoporosis. The best way to put constant, uniform stress on the body is—you guessed it—exercise. Studies have shown that weight training is the most beneficial activity for boosting bone density, with jogging ranking as a close second.

This is not to say you have to beat the four-minute mile or bench-press heavy weights (see Chapter 9) to keep your bones healthy. You just have to stay active. If you're currently a couch potato, begin a modest exercise program—say, brisk walking for half an hour four days a week. As a bonus, regular exercise stimulates the production of natural pain killing substances in the brain called **endorphins,** which enhance mood and fight depression. About thirty minutes of exercise every other day is all you need to improve bone density—but the benefits are so great that once you get started you'll want to do more.

The kind of exercise you choose is important—a weekly swim probably won't do it. Weight-bearing exercise like tennis, running, and strength training requires your skeletal system to support the weight of your body and helps build bone. And don't think that it's ever too late to start—exercise builds bone even after osteoporosis has begun to develop.

Your exercise regimen will depend on your current activity level and your age. If you've been fairly sedentary for forty or fifty years, it's not likely that you'll start jogging eight miles on a daily basis. But you *can* start a weight-bearing exercise program of more modest proportions. Walking is a good start, and you can further enhance the effects by wearing leg and wrist weights, eventually moving up to jogging if you're able. In Chapter 9, we'll show you how to start a complete exercise program, along with tips for training and a list of the best exercises to build healthy bones.

Here are a few simple caveats before you begin:

1. As with any new endeavor, it's best to start slowly and progress gradually to avoid strains, sprains, and injuries that will land you back on the couch.
2. If you've been diagnosed with osteoporosis, stay away from activities that require repetitive bending from the waist, since this can increase the risk of a compression fracture.
3. As always, check with your doctor before starting a new exercise program.

Wolff's Law

The theory that putting stress on bones causes them to form more bone is known as Wolff's law, and it has been a widely accepted theory for almost a hundred years. We also know that *lack* of stress on the skeletal system causes bone loss—one reason why bed rest can be so detrimental, especially in the elderly.

Wolff's law was proven true by the astronauts in the mid-1980s. During spaceflight, they were relatively inactive and their bodies weren't subjected to even the normal forces of gravity that put stress on bones. The results were shocking: these young, healthy men developed osteoporosis in only a short period of time. Once they returned to their daily routines, the osteoporosis disappeared.

Surgical Treatments

It's true that lifestyle changes can prevent and treat osteoporosis, but sometimes medical treatment is necessary—especially in the case of fractures. You should know about these surgical treatments in case you face fractures. If nothing else, reading about surgical treatments is a great motivator to put down that third cup of coffee or jog around the block for five more minutes.

Osteoporosis causes fractures primarily in three locations: the spine, the wrist, and the hip. Wrist fractures, usually caused by a fall, are the easiest to treat. The bones are pushed back into normal position under local anesthesia and the arm is immobilize in a cast for about five weeks. Hip and spinal fractures aren't so simple to repair. The general treatment methods for spinal and hip fractures are as follows:

Fractures of the Spine

Spinal fractures, or compression fractures, are common in people with osteoporosis. In a compression fracture, the vertebra is wedge-shaped and shorter in the front than in the back. To prevent further fractures, the spine has to be temporarily immobilized. A removable plastic brace prevents bending forward and causing further compression of the vertebrae. Usually, braces have to be worn for six weeks. They're extremely uncomfortable, and they obviously limit daily activities—including exercise.

Hip Fractures

The second most common kind of fracture from osteoporosis is a fracture of the hip. There are two distinct types of hip fractures, named for the location in which they occur. The first, an **intertrochanteric fracture,** takes place between two normal bumps on the thigh bone called the greater trochanter and the lesser trochanter. This kind of fracture is usually treated by inserting an L-shaped metal pin into the hip bone and along the outside of the thigh bone. A stainless steel plate is then attached to the outside of the thigh bone to immobilize the area. (See Figures 5-1 and 5-2.) The plate stabilizes the fracture without requiring bed rest—an important factor, since complete immobilization can create serious medical complications like blood clots and congestive heart failure.

• The second type of hip fracture is called a **femoral neck fracture,** in which the top of the femur, known as the femoral neck, is fractured. It's usually necessary to treat a femoral neck fracture by replacing the ball of the hip joint with a prosthesis. The initial procedure is somewhat more involved than the pin-and-plate procedure used for intertrochanteric fractures, but it does allow movement, usually as soon as the day after surgery.

• In both types of hip fracture, movement is crucial—and as soon as possible after the fracture occurs. Usually surgery will be performed either the day of the fracture or the following day. While surgery is risky for elderly people, prolonged bed rest can be even more dangerous. If you're in the elderly group, work with your doctor to get up and about as soon as possible.

Drug Treatments

A number of prescription medications to treat osteoporosis are available. Only four—estrogen, Fosamax, Calcitonin, and Raloxifene—are approved by the Food and Drug Administration (FDA) for use in treating osteoporosis. A handful of other experimental drugs are currently in varying stages of research and approval. Most of these drugs are effective but have serious side effects ranging from blood clots to breast cancer. And in most cases, drugs constitute a lifetime regimen—a serious consideration, since researchers don't know what other kinds of side effects may occur over a period of twenty or thirty years.

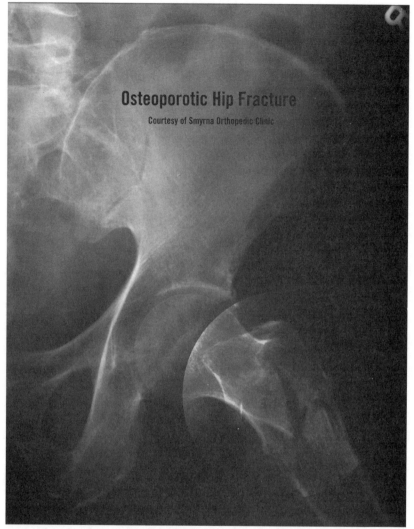

Figure 5-1. Osteoporotic hip fracture. *Courtesy of Smyrna Orthopedic Clinic.*

Estrogen Replacement Therapy (ERT)

While traditional medicine offers many safe and effective procedures for *diagnosing* osteoporosis, *treatment* alternatives are substantially more limited. The most commonly used treatment is estrogen replacement therapy (ERT). Yes, it's effective, but it's also controversial and downright dangerous.

The fact is, estrogen replacement therapy *does* work. It has been proven to reduce the loss of bone mass in postmenopausal women,

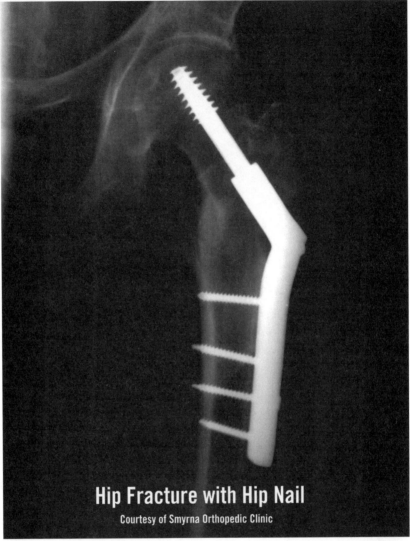

Hip Fracture with Hip Nail

Courtesy of Smyrna Orthopedic Clinic

Figure 5-2. Fracture with hip nail. *Courtesy of Smyrna Orthopedic Clinic.*

and numerous scientific studies have shown that estrogen replacement can reduce the incidence of hip fracture by as much as 50 percent, as well as help prevent heart disease. All these benefits are available—if you're willing to risk a much higher rate of cancer.

While researchers do know that estrogen prevents osteoporosis, they're not exactly sure how it works. Here's the most common theory: estrogen attaches to receptors on osteoclasts and osteoblasts—the cells responsible for bone breakdown and buildup—and alters their activity. In the presence of estrogen, bone is formed, and in the absence of estrogen, bone is lost. The ovaries stop producing estrogen after menopause, so that's when the greatest bone loss occurs— generally during the first five years of menopause.

Estrogen is generally administered in pill form or through injections, vaginal creams, and skin patches. Pills and injections are the most commonly used methods for treating osteoporosis because they deliver much higher levels of estrogen. Vaginal creams can help alleviate some of the effects of menopause like vaginal dryness, but they probably can't deliver enough estrogen to make a substantial difference in the treatment of osteoporosis. Skin patches have become increasingly popular because they're easier to use and can deliver a fair amount of estrogen.

While there are no magic pills, there *are* far safer, natural approaches that are as effective as estrogen. **Ipriflavone,** the new natural supplement we've been hinting at in earlier chapters, works in much the same way as estrogen but without its side effects. We'll talk about ipriflavone in its own chapter later in this book. Meanwhile, here are some reasons why you might want an alternative to estrogen.

- Some studies have shown that women on ERT for ten years have experienced twice the incidence of **breast cancer** of women not on ERT. Other studies have shown a 32 to 36 percent higher risk of breast cancer in women on ERT. But not everyone agrees: some researchers have found no appreciable increase of breast cancer associated with long-term ERT treatment.
- Women on ERT are two to three times more likely to have **blood clots** in the deep veins of the leg. These blood clots can break loose and cause a pulmonary embolism, which can be deadly.
- Many studies in the 1970s were peppered with reports of **endometrial cancer** in women who were taking estrogen alone. Researchers found, however, that when the hormone progesterone was added to the estrogen replacement therapy regimen, the incidence of endometrial cancer dropped dramatically. In other words, if you do opt for ERT, you should be taking progesterone as well.

Studies are now showing that progesterone is as important as estrogen and can significantly reduce the risk of cancer when estrogen replacement therapy is used.

The decision to take ERT is a very individual and personal one. Even the medical community is split: some doctors feel that if diagnostic procedures suggest an increased risk of hip fracture, ERT could be advisable, and ERT may be recommended for women who have had a hysterectomy or those with heart disease. Other doctors feel that it's just not worth the risk, especially since there *are* safer ways to deal with osteoporosis.

If your doctor feels that the risks involved in taking ERT outweigh the risks of osteoporosis, he or she may recommend other prescription medications. Nonhormonal treatment plans can be just as effective as ERT, with fewer side effects. But any synthetic drug has side effects—unlike the natural supplements we'll be talking about in later chapters. If your doctor doesn't know about the natural alternatives to estrogen, like ipriflavone, bring this book to him or her. Ask questions and look for complementary therapies. Remember, it's *your* body and *your* health, and *you* get to make the final decision.

Have We Overlooked Progesterone?

With political and economic factors behind the estrogen campaign, some physicians have looked the other way. With respect to osteoporosis, Dr. John Lee presented the hypothesis that natural progesterone and not estrogen is the missing factor, as published in *Medical Hypothesis* (1991). In a clinical setting, Dr. Lee was able to demonstrate that natural progesterone was extraordinarily effective in reversing the osteoporotic process without the use of estrogen. It seems that progesterone works to influence the bone building process by stimulating osteoblasts independent of estrogen. Others have followed suit. In a 1991 study published in the *Canadian Journal of OB/GYN*, Dr. Prior and others conclude that progesterone is capable of attaching to the osteoblasts and can increase the rate of bone remodeling. Additionally, it seems that adding progesterone to estrogen therapy can significantly enhance the cardioprotective effects of lowering LDL cholesterol ("bad" cholesterol), raise HDL cholesterol ("good" cholesterol), and lower the lipoprotein[a] concentrations that are associated with cardiovascular disease risk.

Have we overlooked the role of natural progesterone? The answer seems to be "yes." Nevertheless, more research needs to be conducted and more physicians need to be willing to review this intriguing work.

Calcitonin

Calcitonin, a hormone made by the thyroid gland, has a direct and positive effect on bone health. As we saw in earlier chapters, calcitonin helps increase absorption of calcium and phosphorus from the blood and boosts bone mineralization. It works by binding to the osteoclasts that break down bone and rendering them ineffective. In the presence of calcitonin, osteoclasts tend to die sooner than they normally would, and calcitonin prevents new osteoclasts from taking their place. The calcitonin used to treat osteoporosis is derived from salmon, and it's extremely effective. Ironically enough, synthetic salmon calcitonin is even more effective in preventing and treating osteoporosis than the calcitonin we make in our own bodies. Studies show that calcitonin:

- Helps reduce bone loss in women even when started more than five years after menopause.
- Significantly reduces the risk of new spine fractures following its use. Some studies show a 30 percent reduction in fractures.
- Can definitely reduce the risk of new fractures by up to 50 percent.
- Creates a sense of well-being, possibly from the stimulation of endorphin production.

Until recently, calcitonin had to be injected—a significant disadvantage. But in 1995, calcitonin became available as a nasal spray. The effects are similar to injectable calcitonin, but a higher dosage is needed in nasal spray form. The spray is easier to administer, and the medication is rapidly absorbed by the mucous membranes in the nasal cavity. In addition, the side effects of injectable calcitonin—primarily nausea and flushing—are significantly reduced using nasal sprays. It's not without its drawbacks, however. Local side effects of calcitonin nasal spray include dryness of the nasal lining, nosebleeds, and itching. In its injectable form, calcitonin can cause nausea, flushing, and diarrhea.

Clinical trials have also shown that calcitonin also seems to have an analgesic effect. Before a full-blown fracture occurs, most people have a number of micro fractures. These minifractures aren't immediately apparent on X rays, but they are extremely painful. Calcitonin has been shown to ease the pain related to microfractures. Researchers aren't sure how calcitonin works in terms of its analgesic effect, but it may be that calcitonin stimulates the formation of endorphins, the body's feel-good chemicals. Other researchers suggest that it's simply a placebo effect. In either case, calcitonin does seem to relieve the pain of microfractures, so how it works may not be so important.

Fosamax

Fosamax is the trade name for a compound called alendronate, one of a large group of compounds called biphosphonates that traditional doctors consider one of the most viable solutions to osteoporosis. Right now, Fosamax is the only nonhormonal preparation for osteoporosis that can be taken in tablet form—and most people would much rather take a tablet every morning than inject themselves.

Biphosphonates, the active ingredients in Fosamax, are a group of compounds that have the ability to attach themselves to minerals. In the body, they bind to the mineral portion of bone and crowd out the osteoclasts, preventing them from functioning in their normal fashion—that is, breaking down bone.

One of the first drugs in the biphosphonate group was called Didronel, used to treat **Paget's disease**—a condition in which bone breakdown and repair are both accelerated and chaotic, with resulting poor bone formation. Researchers have found that Didronel had the fortunate side effect of increasing bone mineralization in people who had suffered a spinal fracture. But because researchers have yet to prove that Didronel can decrease the risk of *repeat* fractures, the drug is approved only for Paget's disease, not for osteoporosis. Fosamax, on the other hand, has been conclusively proven to decrease the incidence of repeat spinal fractures. Other studies have shown that Fosamax:

- Increases bone density in the hip region by as much as 7 percent.
- Helps prevent fractures of both the vertebrae and long bones like the femur.
- Increases bone density by 8 percent in the spine and hip area.
- Decreases the rate of repeat vertebral fractures by 50 percent, after long-term use.
- Decreases the risk of hip fracture by 50 percent after long-term use.

Alendronate can be administered either orally or intravenously. Some studies suggest that intravenous administration, used intermittently every few months, is as effective as daily oral medication. A much lower dose given intravenously over a four-day period has been shown to have the same effect as one year of oral therapy. The oral route, however, is still the preferred method of administration.

Of course, these effects come at a price. Fosamax tends to cause gastrointestinal disturbances, including nausea and constipation, as well as irritation of the esophagus and stomach lining. Another point to consider: Fosamax hasn't been used for long, and it is known to accumulate in the skeleton, so its long-term safety is still in doubt.

Raloxifene

Raloxifene has been proven to stop bone loss and increase bone density without increasing the breast cancer rate as estrogen does. In fact, Raloxifene actually *decreases* the incidence of breast cancer by as much as 58 percent. Raloxifene also lowers cholesterol levels and enhances mood in postmenopausal women. So far, Raloxifene has been used primarily as a preventive measure against osteoporosis and will likely be approved by the FDA for use in treating osteoporosis as well. But it does have side effects, including a substantial increase in hot flashes.

Experimental Drugs

So far, the drugs most frequently used to treat osteoporosis work primarily by inhibiting bone breakdown. But the body fights for equilibrium, and researchers know that, over time, the body will tend to balance itself out. It's possible that bone formation may eventually slow down to equal bone breakdown. In other words, drugs that work only by inhibiting bone breakdown may not be effective over a long period of time. Other treatment modalities that increase bone *formation* instead of, or in addition to, inhibiting bone breakdown are being studied. Some treatments under study are as follows:

• **Sodium fluoride** A compound that, taken orally in very low doses, can stimulate the formation of new bone. Fluoride has not yet been approved by the FDA for treating osteoporosis, but studies are under way, and some are showing promising results. A newly developed, slow-release form of sodium fluoride appears to reduce the risk of fractures in people with osteoporosis, and does so with fewer side effects.

Fluoride increases the number of osteoblasts, the bone builders, and creates fairly dense bone. But one study has shown that sodium fluoride isn't the answer to all the problems related to osteoporosis. In this study, even though fluoride supplement was associated with denser bones, the rate of fractures was about the same. And fluoride appears to create lower-quality bones that tend to be more fragile.

Some research has shown that after fluoride supplementation, the hard portion of the bone that's so important in determining bone strength is lower in mineral density, while the spongy portion of the bone that's important for flexibility has a higher mineral density. Certain studies have even shown that high doses of fluoride can actually increase the risk of fractures from osteoporosis.

As you've no doubt gathered, the use of sodium fluoride to treat osteoporosis is still open to debate, and not least because of its known side effects. Most of these are gastrointestinal in nature, including nausea, vomiting, abdominal pain, and the formation of ulcers. In a handful of studies, fluoride has also been associated with bone cancer.

• **Calcitriol** Technically known as 1,25-dihydroxy-vitamin D, calcitriol is made in the kidney and is the most active and potent form of vitamin D. A synthetic version of calcitriol is sold under the name Rocaltrol and has been approved for use. Rocaltrol stimulates increased absorption of calcium from the intestines and can prevent osteoporosis. But it's rarely used because of its substantial side effects, which include hypercalcemia and resulting kidney stones.

• **Designer Estrogens** When women hit menopause, all kinds of unpleasant symptoms begin—hot flashes, night sweats, and dryness of the vagina and skin. In addition to being remarkably effective in treating osteoporosis, estrogen replacement therapy (ERT) can also alleviate many or most of the symptoms of menopause. But estrogen's side effects can be deadly, so researchers have been scrambling to find adequate substitutes. The results? A class of drugs called designer estrogens.

The interest in designer estrogens was stimulated after an anti-cancer drug known as **tamoxifen** was shown to have the side effect of decreasing the risk of osteoporosis. It seemed like a miracle drug, one that would offer the beneficial effects of estrogen on bone, while protecting against breast cancer. But tamoxifen has some pretty serious side effects, including an increase in the risk of uterine cancer.

• **Tibolone** A type of steroid—also classified as a designer estrogen—that has been proven to stop bone loss and may be useful in the treatment of osteoporosis by slowing the rate of bone breakdown. It's now sold in Europe under the trade name Livial, but it hasn't yet been approved by the FDA for use in the United States. But while Livial may prevent osteoporosis, it also tends to decrease HDL (the "good" cholesterol) levels by as much as 30 percent and increases the risk of heart disease.

Natural Alternatives

Now that we've gone over the most commonly used medications for osteoporosis, along with their potentially dangerous side effects, you are probably eager to hear about a better solution.

The safe and effective alternative is ipriflavone, an estrogen-like compound that prevents and treats osteoporosis without the side effects of drugs.

Studies have shown that ipriflavone not only decreases bone loss but also stimulates new bone formation—a tremendous added benefit, since the most commonly used drugs work only by inhibiting bone breakdown. Since ipriflavone is such a significant breakthrough, we've given it a chapter of its own later.

COMMON DRUGS AND THEIR SIDE EFFECTS

Drug	Action	Side Effect
Estrogen	Can reduce incidence of fractures; enhances osteoblast activity; increases bone density.	Increases risk of breast cancer, endometrial cancer, and blood clots.
Calcitonin	Increases absorption of calcium; inactivates osteoblasts; reduces risk of fractures.	Oral form causes nausea, flushing, and diarrhea; nasal form causes dryness of the nasal lining, nosebleeds, and itching.
Fosamax	Interferes with the function of osteoclasts; reduces risk of fracture; increases bone density.	Causes gastrointestinal disturbances such as nausea and constipation; accumulates in the skeleton; long-term safety is still in question.
Raloxifene	Increases bone density.	Causes hot flashes.
Sodium fluoride	Increases the number of osteoblasts.	Creates poor-quality, fragile bone; can increase the risk of fracture; causes gastrointestinal disturbances and ulcers; may cause bone cancer.

Calcitriol	Increases absorption of calcium.	Causes elevated calcium in the blood, which can result in kidney stones.
Tamoxifen	Has beneficial effects on bone similar to those of estrogen.	Increases risk of uterine cancer.
Tibolone	Slows the rate of bone breakdown.	Decreases HDL levels and increases risk of heart disease.

The Downside of Drugs

Even the most effective drugs have moderate to severe side effects, ranging from mild nausea to breast cancer. While researchers can pinpoint a handful of side effects, they're limited in their ability to predict long-term results: no one knows how long any one person will have to take a given drug to achieve the required result. And as usage increases in amount and duration, more side effects may manifest themselves—side effects that were never noticed in the developmental stages. That's one reason people shy away from experimental drugs. No one really knows what the long-term effects will be, and few people are willing to be the first to find out.

What It All Means

In this chapter, we've gone over some of the more common traditional approaches, but this is by no means a comprehensive list. Remember that traditional medical approaches can—and should—be combined with complementary therapies and appropriate lifestyle changes in diet and exercise. In the next few chapters, we'll talk more about how food, exercise, supplements, and the new nutritional medicines can augment, or even *replace*, traditional medical treatments for osteoporosis, giving the same beneficial results and without the dangerous side effects.

PART THREE

THE
NEW
COMPLEMENTARY
APPROACH

6

DIETARY INFLUENCES ON BONE

We are a society highly aware of nutrition and diet. We measure portions and count calories and are obsessed with the grams of fat and fiber in every bite we put into our mouths. But beyond the much-publicized calcium connection to osteoporosis, few Americans realize the extent to which nutrition influences healthy bones. The truth is, it's not dairy products—or calcium, or vitamin D— alone that will make or break bone health. Other, equally important, dietary factors also come into play.

As with most diseases, osteoporosis is easier to prevent than to treat, so healthy life practices early on are critical in the osteoporosis treatment regimen. Adequate nutrient intake and regular physical activity are significant factors in the development of greater bone mass by the fourth decade of life. Make no bones about it—calcium is absolutely essential for healthy bones. But it's not the *only* factor, nor does it work independently: other dietary factors like sugar and fiber consumption can affect calcium levels in the body. In other words, an extra glass of milk a day alone won't do much in the way of preventing osteoporosis. Basically, everything you put into your mouth—from your morning coffee to your nighttime medications—affects the health of your bones.

The major players in any diet are proteins, carbohydrates, and fats, yet the role of these macronutrients in bone health is frequently overlooked. We know that excess fat is bad for the heart, for instance, but how does it affect bone? Carbohydrates boost energy, but can excess carbohydrates lead to osteoporosis? And while protein is critical for building bones, can too much protein hasten our skeletal demise?

Carbohydrates and Sugars: Sweet Nothings

The new dietary rules exalt a high-carbohydrate diet as the pinnacle of healthy eating, and with good reason. Carbohydrates serve as the chief fuel for energy production in all body processes and keep the body from breaking down protein for fuel. In broad terms, carbohydrates can be divided into two groups: *simple sugars,* like refined white sugar, and *complex carbohydrates,* like those found in vegetables and whole grains. And by no means are these two groups of equal nutritional value.

White sugar is regarded among health purists with the same disdain as cigarettes. Nonetheless, the lure of sweets is so powerful that Americans eat an average of about 150 grams of refined white sugar a day—close to two-thirds of a cup, or the equivalent of fifteen cookies. These statistics bode poorly for bone health: simple sugars increase the excretion of calcium, and there's an inverse relationship between sugar consumption and bone density. In other words, as the amount of sugar intake increases, bone density decreases.

Fiber, an indigestible type of carbohydrate, is also divided into two categories: soluble and insoluble. **Soluble fibers,** found in oats, legumes, apples, and citrus fruits, may enhance the absorption of both calcium and magnesium. By slowing the movement of food through the digestive tract, soluble fiber allows greater absorption of nutrients like the minerals needed for healthy bones. **Insoluble fibers,** found in wheat, wheat bran, flax seed, psyllium husks, and other grains, speed the movement of food through the digestive tract and make calcium *less* available to the body.

And even though we should still eat our grains and greens, some complex carbohydrates contain compounds that aren't necessarily bone-friendly. Phytic acid, found in legumes and the outer husk of cereal grains, binds with calcium to form an insoluble complex that prevents the absorption of calcium. You probably don't need to worry about phytic acid, unless you're eating a lot of beans or whole grains at the same time you're consuming your high-calcium foods. But for those of you who thrive on leafy greens, be forewarned: spinach and certain other vegetables, like beet tops, Swiss chard, and rhubarb, contain high amounts of oxalic acid, which, like phytic acid, binds to calcium and renders it unabsorbable. This certainly doesn't mean you should give up greens. Just eat them at a different meal than your other sources of calcium.

Facts About Fats and Oils

Fat facts have been making headlines for the past ten years. It's well-known that in high amounts or in the wrong proportions, fats and oils contribute to heart disease, cancer, neurological diseases, and other disorders. Less well known is their effect on osteoporosis. In short, excessive consumption of fats and oils can lower calcium levels in the body, thereby contributing to osteoporosis.

Fats and oils possess the same general structure and chemical characteristics but vary in their physical characteristics. Saturated fats, found in animal products, margarine, and tropical oils like coconut oil, are solid at room temperature. Oils (also called unsaturated fats) come from vegetables, nuts, and seeds, and are liquid at room temperature. They have varying effects on calcium levels in the body.

- In large quantities, fats and oils increase calcium excretion and inhibit the absorption of calcium from the digestive tract.
- Saturated fats can bind to calcium and other minerals, and form insoluble compounds that pass through the digestive tract unabsorbed.
- Saturated fats may bind dietary vitamin D, further inhibiting the absorption of calcium and other minerals.
- Heavy fat consumption boosts LDL cholesterol levels, which in turn inhibits the production of a certain enzyme associated with bone formation.

It's the Type of Fat That Matters

Not all fats are off-limits in a bone-healthy diet; some are safer than others. The detrimental effects on bone seem to be associated with saturated fats and certain unsaturated oils, such as corn oil, safflower oil, and soybean oil, in high quantities. These oils enhance the production of inflammatory cytokines, which are damaging to bone, as we saw in the chapter on the bone-immune connection. Other fats may, in fact, have the opposite effect: researchers have shown that monounsaturated fats, like the ones found in olive oil, may actually preserve bone mass and protect against osteoporosis. And Omega-3 fatty acids, found in fish, can also help boost bone health. The best advice? Pass up the butter, please, and stick to olive oil instead.

SOURCES OF SATURATED FATS

Food Source	Percent Saturated Fat
Coconut oil	87
Butter	51
Palm oil	49
Beef tallow	48
Mutton tallow	47
Lard	39
Baking chocolate	30
Chicken fat	30
Shortening	25
Cream cheese	22
Cheddar cheese	21
Processed cheese	20
Beef, ribs	19
Margarine	19
Brazil nuts	17
Peanut oil	17
Lamb chops	16
Soybean oil	14
Olive oil	14
Sour cream	13
Pork sausage	12
Pork chops	11
Hamburger	10

Fatty Acids: A Fishy Story

You listened for years while your mother and the media waxed poetic about milk. Now, studies show that you'll probably want to add a fish dish or two to your diet plan. Fish is high in two types of fatty acids—eicosapentaenoic acid (EPA) and docosahexanoic acid (DHA)—that are especially significant to bone health. EPA and DHA are in a class of compounds commonly known as Omega-3 fatty acids and are found in high concentrations in deepwater fish like tuna, salmon, and swordfish. They also occur in smaller amounts in canola oil, flaxseed oil, and walnut oil.

Of late, Omega-3 fatty acids in general have become recognized for their role in warding off heart disease, and they're also effective in treating inflammatory disorders like arthritis. The anti-inflammatory aspect of Omega-3 fatty acids is relevant to osteoporosis because of the correlation between inflammation and bone metabolism. As we saw in the bone-immune connection chapter, inflammation is a sign that the body is defending itself against microbes or other foreign invaders. Cytokines are one of the many chemicals that regulate inflammation, so when inflammation occurs, cytokine production is stepped up. Certain cytokines, such as interleukin-6 and interleukin-8, stimulate the activity of osteoclasts, which increase bone breakdown. It's no surprise, then, that chronic inflammatory conditions like rheumatoid arthritis are related to a higher risk of osteoporosis.

Studies have shown that two types of Omega-3 fatty acids, EPA and DHA, can help prevent osteoporosis. EPA and DHA supplementation seems to suppress the production of cytokines, which in turn leads to less inflammation. Reduced levels of certain cytokines normalize bone breakdown and preserve bone mineral density. EPA supplementation has an additional benefit: it helps prevent the bone loss associated with the drop in estrogen levels that occurs during menopause.

Sources of Omega-3 Fatty Acids

Cold-Water Fish Oils
- Atlantic cod
- Atlantic salmon
- Bluefish
- Flounder
- Halibut
- Herring
- Mackerel
- Sockeye salmon
- Striped bass
- Tuna

Cooking Oils
- Canola oil
- Evening primrose oil
- Flaxseed oil
- Walnut oil
- Wheat germ oil

Supplements
- Max EPA™ (a source of Omega-3 fatty acids derived from fish)
- Neuromins DHA™ (a source of Omega-3 fatty acids derived from algae, a nonfish, nonanimal food)

Protein: The Good and the Bad

Protein was the first substance to be recognized as a vital part of living tissue. The word itself comes from the Greek word *proteos*, meaning "prime importance." Protein is a critical factor in bone health: it makes up the collagen that reinforces bone, as well as the enzymes that break collagen down. An adequate supply of protein is necessary for bone health, but too much protein can be bad for bones.

The recommended daily allowance of protein is about 63 grams for a 174-pound male and 50 grams per day for a 138-pound female, but Americans are notorious for exceeding these levels. In fact, a protein intake of 100 grams or more per day is not uncommon for the American population—a habit that can be disastrous for bones. When protein is broken down, highly acidic by-products are formed and accumulate in the urine. Since the body strives to maintain a balance between alkaline and acid levels, it mobilizes calcium in the form of bicarbonate, an alkaline compound that can offset increasing acid levels. The calcium that's mobilized is taken from bone. Hence, excessive protein consumption can lead to excessive calcium depletion. Studies have found that:

- Excessive amounts of protein prompt the body to excrete more calcium.
- Raising protein intake from about 50 grams to 150 grams can *double* the amount of calcium excreted.
- Women who consume more than 95 grams of protein a day have a higher risk of forearm fractures than those whose protein intake is less than 68 grams a day

One important note: the *type* of protein consumed may be more important than the *amount*. Women following a vegetarian diet for more than twenty years demonstrated only an 18 percent loss in bone mass by the age of 80, compared to their omnivore counterparts, who experienced a 35 percent decrease—almost twice as high.

A diet high in animal products seems to predispose women to a greater risk for osteoporosis, while a plant-based diet with adequate protein appears to be more conducive to healthy bone growth.

This important finding may have to do with hormonal influences. Researchers have focused their attention on phytoestrogens, a class of hormone-like compounds found in soy products like tofu as well as in whole grain cereals, seeds, berries, and herbs: in other words, foods that are a central component of the typical vegetarian diet. We'll talk in more detail about phytoestrogens in the following section, but first let's take a look at how to calculate your daily protein requirement.

Calculating Protein Requirements

1. Convert your weight in pounds to kilograms by dividing by 2.2
2. Multiply your weight in kilograms by 0.8.
3. Use the answer to determine your protein requirement per day.

The Joy of Soy and Bone Health

There's one easy and effective dietary change you can make in taking care of your bones: add more soy to your diet. Tofu, soy milk, tempeh, and other soy-based foods can actually lower your risk of osteoporosis. Sounds too good to be true? It's not. Studies have shown that certain compounds in soy can actually help build stronger bones. We'll show you ways to add more soy to your diet in the recipe section of this book.

Researchers have become more and more interested in the relationship between bone health and substances called phytoestrogens, or plant estrogens, found primarily in soy. Over the past few years, several major international symposiums have been held to report on the health benefits associated with soy and its active compounds. The consensus? These compounds possess extraordinary healing powers and may play key roles in the prevention of major diseases, including osteoporosis.

Bone Building Phytonutrients at a Glance

- **Phytoestrogen** A type of compound found primarily in plants that has estrogenlike qualities.
- **Isoflavone** One type of phytoestrogen. Soy is a rich source of isoflavones, and it is isoflavones from which ipriflavone, the remarkable new treatment for osteoporosis, is synthesized.
- **Genistein** One type of isoflavone, found only in soy.
- **Daidzein** Another type of isoflavone.

As we noted in the first two chapters, estrogen exerts a protective effect on bone density. Postmenopausal women experiencing a decline in estrogen levels commonly experience an accelerated loss of bone mass. Phytoestrogens act as weaker forms of human estrogen, and may protect against bone loss by acting like estrogen. This is where soy comes in. Besides being one of the richest sources of phytoestrogens, soy is the *only* source of genistein, a type of isoflavone. Much research has shown that genistein and daidzein, another type of isoflavone in soy, can successfully treat osteoporosis and other diseases. One study, for example, showed that genistein was as effective as estrogen in helping to retain bone mass. Genistein also inhibits the actions of a certain enzyme that osteoclasts depend on for their ability to act.

More About Phytoestrogens

Phytoestrogens are plant chemicals that protect plants from fungi, pests, and ultraviolet radiation. These compounds were first identified in the early 1930s, when soybeans and pomegranates were identified as sources of compounds that were structurally similar to estrogens. Interest in phytoestrogens began when researchers noted alterations in the reproductive systems of sheep that fed on certain clovers rich in phytoestrogens. It was later discovered that the effect was attributed to those chemicals in food that exhibited estrogenlike properties. Since then, researchers have identified more than three hundred plants with estrogenic activity. Today, the focus has shifted to sources of phytoestrogens in the human diet, most of which are in soybean products.

Now, here's the catch: even though we know that soy is good for us, Americans have yet to embrace soy-based products in our daily diets. The image of bland white tofu just doesn't click with us. In Japan, the average intake of soy products is about 30 to 50 grams a day. In the United States, the intake hovers somewhere around 3 grams a day. This huge difference in soy intake may explain why, in countries where soy is a main staple of the diet, the rates of osteoporosis and other diseases are much lower than they are in the United States. But even if you're not ready to give up meat yet, perhaps you could try substituting some tofu or tempeh for your burgers and chicken breasts.

What Are Isoflavones?

Isoflavones are natural plant phytoestrogens found in foods (again, like soy), which have been shown to be extraordinarily effective against a number of diseases, including osteoporosis. Researchers of late have been paying more attention to these natural, estrogenlike compounds. Although phytoestrogens in general have been used medicinally for thousands of years, a flurry of research over the past decade has provided much impressive data about the disease-preventive effects of isoflavones. They've been shown to help prevent cancer, heart disease, and other diseases, and can help prevent and treat osteoporosis.

Chemically, isoflavones look very much like the female sex hormone estrogen. In the body, isoflavones are converted into very weak forms of estrogen. Even in their weaker form, they still have powerful disease-preventive effects. Isoflavones, like estrogens, have been shown to preserve bone mass. But unlike estrogen, they're not associated with an increased risk of cancer or other side effects associated with estrogen replacement therapy (ERT). In fact, the isoflavones found in soy are known anticarcinogens and may even *decrease* the risk of cancer.

Isoflavones may be important agents to replace estrogen or to be used in conjunction with estrogen.

Researchers aren't exactly sure how isoflavones work to preserve bone, but theories and speculation abound. In general, it's thought that isoflavones work in essentially the same way as estrogen—by enhancing the activity of osteoblasts to build bone, and decreasing the activity of osteoclasts, which break down bone. We'll talk more about isoflavones and how they work in later chapters.

And for those of you eager to know more immediately, the following table lists the isoflavone content of various soy foods.

THE ISOFLAVONE CONTENT OF SOY FOODS (mg/gram)

Food	Daidzein	Genistein	Glycetein	Total
Roasted soybeans	0.941	1.426	0.294	2.661
Tofu	0.238	0.245	0.049	0.532
Tempeh	0.405	0.422	0.038	0.865
Miso	0.143	0.223	0.023	0.389
Soy hot dog	0.055	0.129	0.052	0.236
Soy bacon	0.026	0.083	0.035	0.144
Tempeh burger	0.095	0.255	0.036	0.386
Tofu yogurt	0.103	0.162	0.017	0.282

Modified from: Anderson, R.L., and W.J. Wolf, *Compositional changes in trypsin inhibitors, phytic acid, saponins, and isoflavones related to soybean processing,* J. Nutr 1995; 125(3): 581–586.

NOTE: For those of you who have not acquired a taste for soy or soy-containing foods, do not despair. There are several excellent dietary supplements on the market that have more than ample levels of the important class of isoflavones. As a matter of fact, you may get substantial levels of isoflavones in a few capsules, tablets or powder as compared to the amount you would need from foods. Look at our resource section in the back of the book for a list of companies that sell soy isoflavone products.

Recommended Resource for Isoflavones: Look for the special registered trademark SoyLife® on the label of your supplement (see resource section). SoyLife® is a registered trademark of Schouten, USA—makers of high quality soy isoflavones and soy concentrates.

Hold the Cheese, Please: Nondairy Sources of Calcium

We all know how important calcium is to bone health. And we also know that dairy products are packed with it. But getting adequate calcium isn't as easy as downing a couple of glasses of milk a day. A hefty portion of our population is allergic to dairy products, and a growing number of vegetarians are giving up milk and cheese altogether. But is it possible to get adequate amounts of calcium from sources other than dairy products?

The dairy-calcium link has been firmly established in our minds by the milk industry's pervasive advertising campaigns. The fact is, however, that one cup of most dark, leafy greens has nearly as much calcium as a cup of milk. Sea vegetables actually have more. It's also known that the protein in dairy products may inhibit calcium absorption. Consider this: in most Asian countries, where dairy products are avoided, where protein consumption is moderate, and where soy products and sea vegetables are abundant, the rate of osteoporosis is significantly lower.

Lots of animal-free foods have enough calcium to make up for milk. Dark leafy greens, broccoli, and sea vegetables are packed with calcium, and they are better absorbed by the body. Studies have shown that the absorption of calcium from kale is 41 percent, compared to a 32 percent absorption rate from milk. Calcium-fortified rice and soy milks have as much calcium and vitamin D per serving as milk. And tofu lovers take heart: soybeans are rich in calcium. Ensuring adequate calcium intake is as easy as adding a serving of tofu, a few handfuls of greens, and a couple of cups of calcium-fortified rice or soy milk to your daily diet. So hold the cheese, please, and try the recipes at the end of this book for better bone health.

THE CALCIUM CONTENT OF SELECTED FOODS

Food	Amount	Calcium (mg)
Wakame (sea vegetable)	½ cup	1700
Agar agar (sea vegetable)	¼ cup	1000
Nori (sea vegetable)	½ cup	600
Kombu (sea vegetable)	¼ cup	500
Sardines with bones	½ cup	500
Sesame seeds	¼ cup	500
Turnip greens, cooked	1 cup	450
Tempeh	1 cup	340
Collard greens, cooked	1 cup	300
Shrimp	1 cup	300
Mackerel with bones	½ cup	300
Milk	1 cup	288
Fortified rice milk	1 cup	280
Fortified soy milk	1 cup	280
Canned red salmon	½ cup	275
Yogurt	1 cup	272
Kale, cooked	1 cup	200
Mustard greens, cooked	1 cup	180

Broccoli	1 cup	178
Almonds	¼ cup	175
Dandelion greens	1 cup	150
Tofu	1 cup	150
Navy beans	1 cup	140
Soybeans	1 cup	130
Raw oysters	½ cup	120
Hazelnuts	¼ cup	115
Pinto beans	1 cup	100
Garbanzo beans	1 cup	95
Cooked quinoa	1 cup	80
Walnuts	¼ cup	70
Sunflower seeds	¼ cup	70
Lima beans	1 cup	60
Black beans	1 cup	60
Lentils	1 cup	50
Romaine lettuce	1 cup	40
Cooked oats	1 cup	40
Mung bean sprouts	1 cup	35
Alfalfa sprouts	1 cup	25
Cooked brown rice	1 cup	20

Calcium: The Finicky Mineral

What about calcium itself? Well, whether your calcium comes from milk or collard greens, one fact is clear: it's a fussy little mineral. Left to its own devices, it won't do its work. In order to be absorbed, it must leave the cooperation of a number of supportive nutrients. To maintain adequate levels of calcium in the blood—thereby reducing the chances that the body will steal reserves from bones—vitamin D and magnesium are necessary. And calcium maintains a delicate balancing act with the mineral phosphorus: when phosphorous levels are excessive, calcium will be excreted. (This is a good reason to avoid high-phosphorous commercial sodas.)

Calcium is so demanding that it refuses to work in the presence of some of the most common components of the traditional healthy diet. Certain kinds of fiber, for example, bind to the mineral and block its absorption. Excess protein also appears to interfere with calcium uptake and can actually increase calcium loss. (This is another reason why dairy may not always be the best source of calcium.) And while spinach has lots of calcium, it also contains a substance called oxalic acid that inhibits the absorption of calcium.

Sodium: Rubbing Salt in Our Wounds

Early civilizations considered salt a priceless commodity, one to be used sparingly and prudently. Today, we put it in everything from toothpaste to tortilla chips. The chemical name for salt is sodium chloride, a substance that's been linked with hypertension and heart disease. What's not as commonly recognized is the link between sodium—which makes up about 40 percent of table salt—and osteoporosis.

Excessive sodium intake boosts the excretion of calcium, resulting in a loss of minerals in bone and an overall decrease in bone strength. Additionally, when researchers examined the effects of salt on bone metabolism, they found that the excretion of hydroxyproline—a chemical that indicates the level of bone break-down—increased with sodium intake. Conversely, hydroxyproline levels (and bone breakdown) were offset with higher calcium intakes. This doesn't mean you have to throw away your salt shaker. Just keep your eye on hidden sources, and shake prudently.

Food Additives That Contain Sodium

- Disodium phosphate
- Monosodium glutamate
- Sodium alginate
- Sodium benzoate
- Sodium hydroxide
- Sodium proprionate
- Sodium sulfite
- Sodium pectinate
- Sodium caseinate
- Sodium bicarbonate

Caffeine: Stimulating More Than Our Nerves

In today's fast paced world, sleep sometimes seems more a luxury than a necessity. Hence, the popularity of coffee in our current climate of movers and shakers. But it's not just in coffee: caffeine is a naturally occurring compound also found in tea, cocoa, and chocolate. It's also hidden in a number of popular nonprescription medications, like pain relievers and cold medications.

The link between calcium and caffeine is intimate and controversial, and the balance between these two substances is delicate. For every cup of coffee consumed, the body's calcium balance—the difference between calcium intake and excretion—becomes negative. If you drink more than a couple of cups of coffee a day, the calcium loss can be substantial, especially for a population that's already consuming too little calcium. Adding milk to your morning coffee can help offset this loss.

The bottom line: drinking too much coffee can cause bone loss and osteoporosis. Excessive caffeine intake is associated with:

- Increased calcium excretion.
- Decreased blood calcium levels.
- Alteration in levels of the hormones that influence bone metabolism.
- Increased parathyroid hormone levels, which stimulates bone breakdown.
- Decreased availability of testosterone, which can lead to a higher risk of male osteoporosis.

The moral of the story? If you're a proud member of the coffee generation, you don't have to turn in your membership card just yet: moderate caffeine consumption (which means a cup or two a day) appears to be safe. But if you're already at risk of accelerated bone loss, take your coffee with milk, and be aware of other sources of caffeine.

CAFFEINE CONTENT

Food Item	Caffeine Content (mg)
Coffee (6 oz)	
Brewed	103
Instant	57
Decaffeinated	2
Cappuccino	75
French flavored	51
Mocha flavored	34
Tea (6 oz)	
Brewed, black	36
Iced, instant	30
Soft Drinks (12 oz)	26–34
Chocolate/Cocoa	
Semisweet	18
Sweet, dark 1.5 oz	27–31
Baker's, 1 oz	57

Milk chocolate, 1.5 oz	9–11
Medications	
Alertness pill (No-Doz/Vivarin)	100–200
Analgesics (Anacin, Excedrin)	35–65

Carbonated Beverages: Hard Facts on Soft Drinks

Cola and other carbonated beverages have assumed center stage at most American gatherings of all ages and stages of life. Can you imagine a summer picnic or barbecue without a cooler full of the bubbly stuff? But soft drinks are hard on health, and worried mothers have long tallied the number of cans their offspring consume. And as if the sugar and caffeine content of soda weren't bad enough, there's more to fret about: phosphorus, in the form of phosphoric acid used as a preservative in most commercial canned sodas, is also implicated in bone loss.

Phosphorus is necessary for proper bone formation and mineralization. Under normal circumstances, it exists in a delicate balance with calcium. This ratio is critical to bone heath, and an excess of either mineral can hinder absorption and blood concentration of the other. When blood phosphorus levels exceed calcium levels, the body responds by stimulating bone breakdown to release calcium into the bloodstream. Since the average American routinely consumes too little calcium and too much phosphorus, calcium levels are often compromised. High levels of phosphorus also suppress blood levels of vitamin D, which is necessary for optimum calcium absorption. (And remember that sugar and caffeine, primary ingredients in sodas, are also bad for your bones.)

While other foods we've discussed are necessary to some degree, there's no redeeming value in soft drinks at any level of intake. They're nutritional "black holes" at best, and harmful at worst. Studies have shown a strong association between cola intake and increased risk of bone fractures in young girls, a phenomenon which was reversed by increasing calcium intake. Nor is cola the only villain: other soft drinks can also tip the calcium-phosphorous ratio in an unfavorable direction. Meat, dairy products, and fish also have high levels of phosphorous. And as the intake of soda continues to grow, the consumption of healthy beverages like water, juice, and milk decreases. These chemical cocktails may be the life of the party, but they can be the death of your bones.

Alcohol: An Argument for Sobriety

Now that we've seen what's wrong with soft drinks, what about *hard* drinks? It's probably no surprise that the news isn't necessarily good. As with most things, moderation is the key. A modest amount of alcohol—up to seven ounces per week, or two glasses of wine—may be conducive to bone formation, possibly by augmenting estrogen levels, but excessive amounts are a known risk factor for osteoporosis. Studies have shown that alcoholic men have a depressed rate of bone formation, along with an increased rate of bone breakdown. Additionally, alcoholic men are more likely to have fractures related to osteoporosis.

Alcohol has a variety of both direct and indirect effects that can impair bone health and lead to osteoporosis:

- Chronic, excessive alcohol intake stimulates the action of *osteoclasts,* which increase bone breakdown.
- Excessive alcohol consumption boosts the excretion of magnesium, one of the minerals necessary for healthy bones.
- Nutrient deficiencies are common in heavy drinkers, and these can further contribute to the development of osteoporosis.
- Excessive alcohol intake can damage the liver. Since the liver plays an integral part in activating vitamin D—which helps boost calcium absorption—prolonged heavy drinking may mean less calcium incorporated into your bones.

While a glass or two of wine a week probably won't damage your bones, moderation is paramount. And even though a little alcohol may boost bone building, you're probably better off toasting with fruit juice and mineral water spritzers anyway.

Medications: Health Care's Double-Edged Sword

Science has given us the ability to produce medications with greater specificity and potency for a variety of afflictions, and countless lives have been saved by modern medicine. But a magic pill with no side effects has yet to be discovered, and drugs that are intended to cure one condition may cause another. The gamut of potential side effects runs from mild stomach upset to permanent organ failure, and includes osteoporosis. And while medicine isn't food, it *is* a dietary factor that's worth consideration—especially in light of the sometimes cavalier attitude toward drug treatment for even the mildest complaints. Let's look at some of the drugs that have the strongest effects on osteoporosis.

• **Corticosteriods** Cortisol, corticosterone, cortison, and hydrocortisone are a group of chemicals classified as glucocorticoids or corticosteroids. Their anti-inflammatory properties make them useful therapeutic agents for a number of diseases, including rheumatoid arthritis. But the long-term side effects, especially with regard to bone health, greatly limit their clinical application. Corticosteroids are associated with an increased risk of osteoporosis in 50 percent of people on long-term therapy.

In the presence of corticosteroids, calcium absorption and osteoblast activity decrease, while calcium excretion increases. The net results are a negative calcium balance, increased bone breakdown, and ensuing bone loss. Corticosteroid therapy may aggravate bone loss in men by decreasing testosterone levels, which are involved in bone formation. While corticosteroids, like most drugs, do have their place, many people on conventional corticosteroid therapy may be on an inappropriate regimen. Other natural substances are available to treat immune disorders like rheumatoid arthritis, as we discussed at the end of Chapter 2.

• **Thyroid hormone** Thyroid hormone therapy has been successfully used to treat hypothyroidism (a decreased activity of the thyroid gland) and goiter (noncancerous growths of the thyroid gland) for more than ninety years. Abnormal growth or enlargement of the thyroid gland is a characteristic of goiters and cancer. Excess thyroid medication decreases blood levels of thyrotropin, the hormone that's responsible for abnormal thyroid gland growth. Thyroid hormone therapy isn't without its disadvantages and has been linked to osteoporosis. Again, older women are the highest-risk group: they're two to ten times as likely as men to develop thyroid disorders and receive thyroid hormone therapy, and they're also the group most affected by osteoporosis.

Prolonged thyroid hormone treatment may lead to a significant loss of calcium from the bones, increasing the risk of fractures in the spine, hip, and wrists. Thyroid hormone directly affects osteoblasts, stimulating them to release cytokines that then prompt osteoclasts to break down bone. Patients taking more than 200 micrograms of thyroid hormone may have significantly lower bone mineral densities than those taking fewer than 200 micrograms. If you're on this hormone long term, make sure your doctor plans to monitor your bone health on a regular basis.

• **Anticoagulants** As the name implies, anticoagulants prevent blood coagulation (or blood clots) and are used primarily in surgery, during dialysis, and to reduce the risk of stroke and heart attack. In 1963 heparin, a popular and widely used anticoagulant, was speculated as being a possible cause of osteoporosis in those undergoing long-term therapy.

Heparin is available in three forms: low molecular weight, conventional, and high molecular weight. Research has demonstrated that bone loss is greatest in people taking conventional and high-molecular-weight heparin, although the reasons aren't yet known. The action of parathyroid hormone may actually be enhanced by heparin, thus increasing bone resorption and bone loss.

• **Antacids** One of the favorite fast remedies for indigestion, antacids typically contain aluminum, magnesium, and calcium, or a combination of these. They work by decreasing stomach acidity. While this may sound (and feel) good, chronic and prolonged intake may decrease mineral availability. During digestion, the acidic environment of the stomach is critical to allow minerals to be absorbed properly. Antacids hinder absorption by reducing acidity. And, contrary to current advertising campaigns, calcium carbonate—a popular antacid base—doesn't necessarily provide adequate calcium supplementation because of its effects on stomach acid. Another factor: many antacids contain aluminum, which physically binds to minerals and renders them useless. Have you guessed by now that Tums® probably isn't a great source of calcium?

What It All Means

Like every cell, tissue, and organ in the body, bone is diet-dependent, and we have the opportunity to ensure better bones through what we eat and don't eat. Bone, our nutrient bank of minerals, is just like any other bank: the more deposits and the fewer withdrawals you make now, the more you'll have later in life.

We've gone over a lot of dietary factors involved in osteoporosis. But this is still by no means a comprehensive list; the foods and medications noted here are only a few of the factors relevant to bone health. Everything we eat, drink, or swallow alters our bodies, invoking changes for either good or bad. In the next chapter, we'll talk about ways to supplement your diet for better bone health.

7

NUTRITIONAL SUPPLEMENTS FOR HEALTHY BONES

In the preceding chapter, we talked about dietary changes you can make to help build stronger bones. But even the best diet may need some supplementation. Doctors and the modern medical community seem to have developed a veritable calcium fixation, while the many other vitamins, minerals, and trace minerals crucial for normal growth and development of bone are largely ignored. It's important to remember that osteoporosis is a disease that involves both mineral and protein components of bone, and that the protein portion of bone needs nutrients far different from the traditionally prescribed minerals. In this chapter, we'll talk about calcium—and how that can help prevent and treat osteoporosis.

Calcium

Calcium is the most abundant mineral in the body, and most of it—about 99 percent—is deposited in bone. There's no doubt that calcium is a fundamental player in preventing and treating osteoporosis. Numerous studies have shown that calcium supplementation, at levels of 1000 mg to 1500 mg a day, can help reduce bone loss by 30 to 50 percent. A 1998 study published in the prestigious *Calcified Tissue International* journal showed that calcium supplementation at levels of 1000 mg a day suppressed bone breakdown, probably by decreasing parathyroid hormone (PTH) secretion. But take note: in some cases of osteoporosis, there's no evidence of calcium depletion. In other words, even if you take your calcium supplements faithfully, you're not necessarily free and clear. Calcium supplementation is only one substance in a whole range of factors affecting bone health and osteoporosis.

As for prevention, calcium (along with other nutrients) is essential. Low calcium intake during growth phases can contribute to low bone mass by limiting the stores of calcium available to build bone. Increased calcium intake during adolescence can help build bone mass early in life, and the mineral stores laid down in the teen years will ultimately decrease the risk of osteoporosis in later years. So don't wait until you've reached the treatment stage. If you're in your teens, be aware of your calcium intake, and if you're a mother, make sure your daughters get the proper amount of calcium, from both dietary and supplemental sources.

Not for Women Only

In a study performed at the Department of Internal Medicine at the University of Vienna, men who showed signs of vertebral osteoporosis were given 1000 mg a day of calcium, plus calcitonin. After twelve months of treatment, the calcium-and-calcitonin combination resulted in significantly increased bone density of the vertebrae and thigh bones. Additionally, a 1997 study in the *New England Journal of Medicine* showed that inadequate intake of calcium and vitamin D may contribute to the high prevalence of osteoporosis among men as well as women.

Drink Up! Calcium in Mineral Water

As Americans worry more about saturated fat, lactose intolerance, and unhealthy additives in milk, the consumption of dairy products has decreased. At the same time, we're drinking lots more bottled mineral water—a trend that may bode well for bone health. Using studies from the Department of Internal Medicine at the University of California, Davis, researchers found that many bottled mineral waters have high concentrations of calcium and that the calcium in water is absorbed as well or better than the calicum in milk.

This is pretty exciting news—especially if you're not a big dairy fan. These findings were confirmed by European studies, which found that mineral water can be a good supplemental source of calcium. Bottled mineral waters do vary widely in calcium content, however, so check the mineral content on the label of your favorite brand or call the company and ask for a current analysis.

Here is a list of bottled mineral waters that contain calcium. The levels may vary slightly from batch to batch, but most have consistent levels of calcium and other minerals.

Bottled Mineral Water	Source
Colfax Mineral Water	*Colfax, Iowa*
Crystal Geyser	*California*
Evian	*France*
Mountain Valley	*Arkansas*
Naya	*Canada*
Perrier	*France*
Swiss Alp Water	*Switzerland*
Vittel	*France*

The Secrets of Efficient Calcium Absorption

Remember that calcium is helpful to bone health only if you absorb it properly. You can take as many calcium supplements as you want, but if they're not digested and assimilated by the body, you're just throwing your money away and giving yourself a false sense of security. Several factors affect how well the body absorbs calcium. As we age, our digestion becomes less efficient, and the amount of calcium absorbed in the digestive tract decreases. The form in which you take a calcium supplement is also crucial. And Tums® is not the answer. Calcium carbonate—the form of calcium found in Tums®—does have the highest percentage of elemental calcium, but it's poorly absorbed. Studies show that people with decreased stomach acid absorb only about 4 percent of the calcium in its calcium carbonate state, compared to an absorption rate of nearly 50 percent from calcium citrate. And you get what you pay for: inexpensive, generic supplements that offer calcium derived from bone meal and dolomite have a higher content of lead (a known toxin) and aren't absorbed by the body well.

Here are some other tips to remember when you're taking calcium supplements:

- For optimal absorption, calcium should be *chelated,* a procedure that typically involves binding the mineral to an amino acid or carbohydrate so that it's more available to the body. Look for chelated forms of calcium citrate and calcium glycinate.
- Calcium supplements taken in the evening are more likely to reduce bone breakdown. Researchers found that when calcium supplements were taken in the evening, the signs of bone breakdown were significantly reduced. Calcium taken during the day had no significant effect on bone breakdown. For the best results,

take about two-thirds of your daily dose of calcium with your dinner meal or evening snack.

- Don't worry about kidney stone formation, as long as you're taking the right dosage and form of calcium. If you're taking calcium citrate, the citrate part will help prevent stone formation.
- Choose your supplements based on reputation, not price. Reputable manufacturers test their raw materials and finished product for lead, and should be able to tell you whether their products contain lead and how much. If you're not sure, call the manufacturer and ask for the assay results for the lot number you find on your bottle. If they don't have it or won't give it to you, change brands.
- Don't gulp a handful of pills all at once. Dividing your dose of calcium so that you're taking it throughout the day (with meals) and at bedtime will allow your body to absorb and use more calcium. Calcium supplements should be taken with meals to boost their absorption.
- Certain substances can hinder the absorption of calcium. These include zinc supplements, coffee, alcohol, and antacids. If you're using any of these, don't take your calcium supplements at the same time.
- Some foods—including spinach, Swiss chard, and whole wheat or high-fiber cereals—bind to calcium and render it unabsorbable. This doesn't mean you can't have spinach or bran cereals. Just take your calcium supplements at a different meal.
- When you're figuring out how much calcium to take in supplement form, take into consideration how much you get in your diet. If you're an adult with osteoporosis, 1500 mg a day of calcium from food and supplements is plenty. If you're taking ipriflavone, you'll only need about 1000 mg of calcium daily.

Magnesium

Bone is a big warehouse for calcium. It also houses stores of magnesium, a mineral that's critical in the maintenance of bone. Magnesium influences bone health through its effects on hormones and other factors that regulate bone metabolism. It regulates the transport of calcium; a magnesium deficiency can adversely affect all phases of bone breakdown and buildup. In short, magnesium is essential to bone health because it:

- Activates bone-building osteoblasts.
- Increases soft-bone mineralization density.

- Enhances sensitivity of bone tissue to PTH and active vitamin D.
- Facilitates the normal functioning of the parathyroid glands.
- Facilitates the transport of calcium in and out of bone.

In some cases, where calcium intake is sufficient, magnesium supplementation may be even more important than calcium supplementation.

People with osteoporosis generally show signs of magnesium deficiency, and researchers believe that magnesium depletion contributes to osteoporosis. Studies have proven that magnesium has a definite effect on bone health, especially on soft bone—the kind of bone primarily affected in postmenopausal osteoporosis. Here are some of the more interesting findings:

- Researchers have found that emphasizing magnesium instead of calcium in postmenopausal women on estrogen therapy boosted bone mineral density in soft-bone tissue.
- A two-year study at the Sackler Faculty of Medicine in Israel found that magnesium supplementation significantly increased soft-bone density.
- In a 1995 study, published in *Nutrition Reviews*, investigators gave magnesium to postmenopausal women. After two years, magnesium therapy positively influenced bone density and helped to prevent fractures.
- A study published in *Osteoporosis International* in 1996 showed increased bone density and PTH levels after magnesium therapy in people suffering from a diminished ability to absorb nutrients

For a long time it was believed that a high intake of calcium would interfere with magnesium absorption and have an adverse effect on bone health. This long-standing concept was challenged in a 1996 *American Journal of Clinical Nutrition* article, which reported that the magnesium balance of adolescent females who consumed a combined daily total of either 1667 mg or 667 mg of calcium from dietary and supplemental sources was not affected. These findings were further validated in a 1997 study at Purdue University, when researchers also found that high calcium intake did not alter magnesium balance in adolescent females.

On the other hand, we do know that standard treatments for osteoporosis—which include estrogen and high doses of calcium—may have a role in decreasing blood levels of magnesium. Since both excess calcium or estrogen decrease magnesium, the common recommendation for an appropriate calcium-to-magnesium ratio is 2:1. And since magnesium is turning out to be as essential as calcium, it's important to ensure that you get enough magnesium every day, especially if you already have osteoporosis. (For some conditions, such as arthritis and heart disease, the level of magnesium may need to be even higher than calcium. In such cases, it's wise to check with a progressive nutritionist to determine the appropriate calcium/magnesium ratio.)

As with all mineral supplements, chelated forms of magnesium are best. Studies have shown that chelated magnesium citrate and magnesium glycinate are better absorbed and used by the body than inorganic magnesium oxide forms. Magnesium citrate has the added bonus of helping to prevent calcium-stone formation in the kidneys. Magnesium glycinate runs a close second as the best choice. How much magnesium you need depends in part on how much calcium you're getting, since the two minerals should exist in a two-to-one ratio. In other words, if you're taking 1000 mg a day of calcium, you need at least 500 mg of magnesium daily. Since high single doses of magnesium may cause diarrhea, it's best to distribute your total amount throughout the day—about 200 mg with food three or four times a day.

Food Sources of Magnesium

- Brown rice
- Buckwheat
- Corn
- Dandelion greens
- Dark green vegetables
- Legumes
- Nuts (almond, cashew, Brazil)
- Rye
- Seeds (sunflowers, sesame, pumpkin)
- Wheat germ/bran
- Whole grain cereals

Vitamin D

Vitamin D is one of the most important regulators of calcium. It's essential for enhancing calcium absorption in the intestine and decreasing the excretion of calcium in the kidneys. And vitamin D supplementation is backed by a wealth of data illustrating its importance in bone mineralization and its efficacy in treating osteo-porosis.

Sunlight Exposure and Vitamin D

Sunlight exposure
Ultraviolet rays penetrate skin
Cholesterol (dehydrocholesterol) Precholecalciferol Cholecalciferol
▼
Dietary vitamin D   (transformed in the liver)
25-dihydroxyvitamin D
▼
(final transformation in the kidney
to the active form)
1,25-dihydroxyvitamin D

The major function of the active form of vitamin D is to keep the body's blood levels of calcium in the ranges needed to maintain essential cellular functions and to promote bone mineralization. It's well known that women with postmenopausal osteoporosis show some degree of decreased calcium absorption and commonly have low blood levels of vitamin D. Supplementation with vitamin D can help the body absorb calcium better and may have positive effects on bone formation.

Studies have also shown that treating vitamin D deficiency with supplements can significantly reduce the number of hip fractures in people with osteoporosis. A study reported in the *American Journal of Clinical Nutrition* in 1995 offers a case in point. In a double-blind, two-year trial, researchers increased vitamin D intake to 700 IU (the RDA is 200 IU) in a group of postmenopausal women. They found that 200 IU of vitamin D wasn't as effective in decreasing bone loss from the hip as 700 IU. Other research has yielded similar results. In a 1997 study published in the *New England Journal of Medicine*, researchers evaluated the effect of calcium and vitamin D on bone density in both men and women sixty-five years old or older. After three years, the people who took 700 IU of vitamin D and 500 mg of calcium every day had significant increases in bone density.

So how much should *you* take? You may think that, because you can manufacture vitamin D from the sun, you're not at any risk of deficiency. This may not be the case. All kinds of factors—including seasonal changes, differences in climate, and the amount of time spent outside—affect the amount of sun we get and, consequently, how much vitamin D we can make on our own. Aging is another factor: as we get older, our bodies are less efficient at manufacturing vitamin D from the sun. Add to that the fact that older people tend to spend less time outdoors, and you can understand that vitamin D deficiency isn't uncommon. It's likely that this deficiency significantly contributes to decreased calcium absorption—and a corresponding acceleration of bone loss and increased risk of hip fracture.

The current RDA for vitamin D is 200 IU, but this is a maintenance level and isn't nearly enough to have therapeutic value. But more isn't necessarily better: too much vitamin D can be toxic. At very high doses, side effects such as hypercalcemia (excess levels of calcium in the blood), calcification of soft tissue, and kidney stones have been reported. In general, 400 IU to 800 IU is considered effective, and dosages exceeding this amount don't impart any greater benefit. The best forms of supplemental vitamin D are vitamin D_2 (ergocalciferol) and vitamin D_3 (cholecalciferol). The naturally occurring vitamin D_3 is preferred over vitamin D_2. Another note: stay away from the new fat-replacement product called Olestra and all foods containing it. Olestra has been shown to decrease absorption and blood levels of vitamin D as well as other essential nutrients.

Food Sources of Vitamin D

- Butter and margarine
- Cheese
- Egg yolk
- Fish liver oils
- Fortified cereals and breads
- Fortified milk
- Herring
- Mackerel
- Oysters
- Salmon

Vitamin K

Vitamin K is a term used to describe a group of similar compounds which include K_1 (phylloquinone), derived exclusively from food; K_2 (menaquinone), made from bacteria in the intestines; and K_3

(menadione), a synthetic compound. Once thought only to influence the clotting of blood, vitamin K is now emerging as an important part of the total nutritional plan for treating osteoporosis.

Both hard and soft bone contain substantial concentrations of vitamin K. It acts as a cofactor in synthesizing osteocalcin, an important compound involved in bone calcification. Osteocalcin, the major noncollagen protein produced by bone building osteoblasts, is believed to be involved in the very first steps of mineralizing bone tissue.

In elderly people, a form of osteocalcin that binds to bone—and affects bone mineralization—is generally low, but can be increased with vitamin K supplementation. Decreased blood levels of this osteocalcin have been reported in postmenopausal women and those with hip fracture and may indicate vitamin K inadequacy. Some studies have suggested that vitamin K deficiency is one of the risk factors for developing osteoporosis. Here are some other important findings:

• Vitamin K supplementation has been shown to increase bone mineral density in women with vertebral compression fracture as a result of osteoporosis.
• Bone formation increases in postmenopausal women who take supplemental vitamin K.
• In men, decreased levels of vitamin D and vitamin K are associated with the development of osteopenia, another bone disorder.
• Postmenopausal women with low bone density have lower levels of vitamin K than women with normal bone density.

Since 60 to 70 percent of the daily dietary intake of vitamin K is excreted, the body needs a continuous daily supply to maintain adequate levels. The recommended dosage is 150 mcg a day with meals, in addition to the amounts found commonly in the diet. One note of caution, however: if you're on an anticoagulant (blood thinning) medication, you should check with your health care practitioner before you begin supplementing your diet with vitamin K.

Food Sources of Vitamin K

• Broccoli
• Brussels sprouts
• Cauliflower
• Chick peas

- Dairy products
- Eggs
- Kale
- Seeds
- Vegetable oils (olive, canola)

Four Essential Trace Elements

Boron

The need for boron in the human body has been a topic of debate for some fifty years. It wasn't until 1980 that sufficient evidence implicated boron as an essential trace element in animals and humans. Now, research has suggested that boron plays a role in bone metabolism and is most likely associated with its interactions and ability to activate certain vitamins, minerals, and hormones important to bone.

Boron is necessary for the conversion of vitamin D into its active form. This is one of the reasons why boron deficiency has been shown to affect calcium metabolism and bone formation. Studies have shown that boron deprivation causes alterations in calcium metabolism that are bad for bone formation and maintenance. Boron seems to interact with calcium through some mechanism that's not yet understood. Boron not only reduces the loss of calcium from bones, but also increases the levels of active estrogen in the body—a necessary component for bone health. Boron is also needed to activate both estrogen and vitamin D. And a deficiency of boron seems to be associated with an increased risk for postmenopausal bone loss.

Because of the way it works, boron may be an effective therapy for postmenopausal women. In a 1997 study at the United States Department of Agriculture, postmenopausal women who took 3 mg of boron a day showed decreased excretion of calcium and magnesium. The study also implicates boron as an important nutrient that decreases oxalate in the urine and may be important in the control of kidney stone formation. Additionally, boron supplementation markedly increased blood concentrations of a substance called 17-beta-estradiol—an active form of estrogen—and may mimic some of the effects of estrogen on calcium metabolism.

Fruits and vegetables are the main dietary sources of boron, but these food sources only reflect the amount of boron that's in the soil, so they're subject to great fluctuations. It is estimated that the average American intake of boron is approximately 1.7 mg to 7 mg a day, but no one knows whether this intake is optimal. In the meantime, based on scientific studies, the recommended level of supplementation is 3 mg to 5 mg daily, taken with meals.

Food Sources of Boron

- Apples
- Beet greens
- Broccoli
- Cabbage
- Cherries
- Grapes
- Legumes
- Nuts
- Peaches
- Pears

Silicon

Although no one has yet explained silicon's exact biological role, we do know that this trace mineral is important for the proper growth and maintenance of skin, hair, ligaments, tendons, and bone. Silicon is required for the formation of collagen in bone, cartilage, and other connective tissues. And laboratory experiments have demonstrated that silicon is essential for the normal skeletal growth by playing a role in the initial stages of bone development when the protein matrix is constructed.

Some studies suggest that silicon may also increase the rate of bone mineralization. Additional research has shown that silica plays an important role in the formation of apatite crystal, the primary constituent in bone. In a 1993 study at the Center Hospital of Toulon, France, researchers evaluated the effects of silicon, fluoride, magnesium, and etidrodronate on bone mineral density in women with osteoporosis. After a year, women who received silicon supplementation showed a significant increase in bone mass density of the thigh bone.

Because silicon is found primarily in whole, unprocessed foods, the modern American diet has marginal levels of this important substance. Processing techniques strip away the silicon content of many foods, particularly whole grains and cereals. So emphasis on foods high in silicon and the use of supplements is an important part of the nutritional protocol. While there is no RDA for silicon, it is estimated that average daily intakes range from 20 mg to 50 mg. Supplements of the herb horsetail and certain algae should be added to your daily routine. The recommended amount for treating osteoporosis, based on scientific studies, is 25 mg to 50 mg a day, taken with meals.

Food Sources of Silicon

- Asparagus
- Cabbage
- Cucumbers
- Dandelion greens
- Lettuce
- Mustard greens
- Olives
- Parsnips
- Radishes
- White onions
- Whole grains (rice and oats)

Zinc

About 2 grams of zinc are scattered throughout the body, with the highest concentrations in the prostate, eyes, liver, and bone tissue. Zinc is an important player in preventing osteoporosis. Zinc regulates the secretion of calcitonin from the thyroid gland and influences bone turnover. Studies have shown that women with osteoporosis excrete more zinc, which indicates a need for more zinc intake. In one study, researchers evaluated levels of zinc in postmenopausal women, the group most likely to develop osteoporosis. The study found a significant increase in the loss of zinc in postmenopausal women compared to the control group, and suggested that zinc is an important marker of osteoporosis, since its elimination is related to bone turnover.

Maintaining adequate zinc levels is important in traditional treatments of osteoporosis. In a 1996 study, published in the journal *Obstetrics and Gynecology,* researchers evaluated the effects of estrogen replacement therapy (ERT) on zinc levels in postmenopausal women. The study found that zinc loss is associated with decreased bone mineral density in women with osteoporosis. It seems that estrogen is a factor in zinc loss.

It's possible that high calcium intake may interfere with the body's ability to use zinc, but studies show conflicting results. In a 1997 study at the Bone and Mineral Metabolism Laboratory at Ohio State University, researchers found that calcium intake up to 1500 mg daily did not have adverse effects on the body's ability to use zinc. On the other hand, a 1997 study at the Mineral Bioavailability Laboratory at Tufts University showed opposite results: in post-menopausal women, calcium supplements significantly reduced the absorption of zinc absorption. Including additional zinc with calcium supplements offset the detrimental effect of calcium on zinc absorption. The best advice? To offset any possible interference of its absorption by calcium, take 30 mg to 60 mg a day of zinc in its most absorbable, chelated forms: zinc glycinate, zinc picolinate, and zinc citrate. Also, be aware that the absorption of zinc, like calcium, can be inhibited by certain foods. These include legumes, whole grain cereals and breads, wheat bran, and brown rice. For maximum absorption, take your zinc at a different meal.

Food Sources of Zinc

- Brazil nuts
- Oats
- Oysters
- Peanuts
- Pecans
- Pumpkin seeds
- Rye
- Split peas

Copper

Copper is an abundant trace mineral in the body, and about 19 percent of it is contained within the skeletal system. It's responsible for immune function, artery function, protection against oxidative and inflammatory disease, and bone health. A deficiency of copper—which can occur from malnutrition or malabsorption—may compromise bone health.

Copper is essential for the normal growth and development of the skeleton. Because it is found in such minute amounts within bone, copper is considered more important functionally than structurally. Copper affects bone metabolism in two important ways: (1) it induces low bone turnover by suppressing the activity of both osteoblasts (bone builders) and osteoclasts (bone breakers); (2) it helps build bone by contributing to the construction of the protein matrix.

In supplementing with copper, it's critical to pay attention to the zinc-to-copper ratio, since zinc competes with copper for absorption. Ratios of ten or fifteen parts zinc to one part copper are recommended by most experts, but it's not a good idea to exceed 50 mg of zinc for a long period of time. A daily dietary intake of 2 mg to 3 mg a day of copper is a safe bet. As with all minerals, a chelated form is advised. These include copper glycinate, copper gluconate, or copper citrate. Again, be aware of certain foods that can interfere with the absorption of copper, including legumes, whole grain cereals and breads, wheat bran, and brown rice. Again, if your meal is heavy in any of these substances, take copper supplements at a different time.

Food Sources of Copper

- Buckwheat
- Crab
- Liver
- Mushrooms
- Peanut butter
- Seeds and nuts
- Split peas
- Vegetable oils (sunflower, olive)

Vitamin C: Another New Player

While many other nutrients have well-established roles in bone health, vitamin C is just beginning to be recognized as a major player. A 1997 study published in the *Journal of Epidemiology and Community Health* evaluated the difference between dietary and supplemental vitamin C. The study showed that postmenopausal women who took vitamin C supplements for more than ten years had a higher bone mass density than women who did not take any vitamin C. Oddly enough, frequent intake of foods rich in vitamin C was not associated with increasing bone mass density. In short, dietary vitamin C doesn't seem to be associated with bone health, but supplements do. The general recommendation is 500 mg to 1000 mg of vitamin C as calcium ascorbate (buffered form). Higher doses may be used under the guidance of your health care practitioner.

Homocysteine and Osteoporosis

Homocysteine is a harmful substance that has been implicated in the development of atherosclerosis and other diseases, including osteoporosis. In the body, the amino acid methionine is converted to homocysteine, which is then converted back to methionine, or is further converted to another amino acid called cysteine. In some people, that conversion doesn't take place. The conversion of harmful homocysteine back to harmless methionine or cysteine requires several key nutrients, including folic acid, vitamin B_{12}, and vitamin B_6.

$$METHIONINE \rightleftarrows HOMOCYSTEINE \rightarrow CYSTEINE$$

FOLIC ACID   VITAMIN B_6
VITAMIN B_{12}

As you can see, these three B vitamins—folic acid, B_{12}, and B_6—are necessary to convert harmful homocysteine into harmless amino acids.

What does all this have to do with osteoporosis? In one study, homocysteine levels were measured in groups of men, premenopausal women, and postmenopausal women. All were given excessive amounts of methionine, and the body's ability to convert homocysteine back to methionine or to cysteine was evaluated. Researchers found that the postmenopausal women had significantly higher levels of homocysteine than the other groups. Since homocysteine is thought to interfere with proper bone formation, the researchers speculated that elevated levels may contribute to postmenopausal atherosclerosis and osteoporosis.

The following supplements can lower homocysteine levels in the body. There are now homocysteine-reducing formulas that contain all three in a single dose:

- Vitamin B_6: 25 to 50 mg daily with meals
- Folic Acid: 400 mcg daily with meals
- Vitamin B_{12}: 200 mcg daily with meals

Colloidal Minerals—Buyer Beware

Over the past few years, an aggressive marketing campaign riddled with inaccurate and misleading information has popularized colloidal minerals in the dietary supplement market. Unfortunately, many unfounded claims have been made for these products which lack scientific support. They may actually be dangerous to your health. Basically, colloidal minerals are nothing more than mixtures of clays and water. (That's right—the stuff you put on your face!)

To set the record straight: colloidal minerals are not absorbed better in the intestine than chelated minerals. Indeed, extensive scientific and medical literature searches have failed to uncover any studies that support *any* claims made for colloidal minerals. Worse yet, these colloidal mineral clay solutions contain aluminum and other heavy metals that are known to be toxic to your brain, kidneys, liver, and immune system. In a 1977 study published in the *American Journal of Natural Medicine*, Dr. Alex Schauss reported that some of the colloidal mineral products tested contained high levels of aluminum that ranged from 1800 to 4400 ppm (parts per million), compared to similar foods, that generally contain no more than 10 ppm. Also, some of the colloidal mineral products contained 1300 to 22,000 ppm of sodium, which means that hypertensive people should exercise caution.

The bottom line is this: the variability of these products, their potential heavy-metal toxicity, and their lack of safety and efficacy warrant that you *avoid them*. Stick with the proven, safe, and effective chelated mineral products recommended in this chapter.

What It All Means

Preventing and treating osteoporosis isn't as simple as taking a couple of Tums®—or even a high-quality calcium supplement—every day. A range of other factors comes into play, as we've seen in earlier chapters. Nor is calcium the final word in bone-healthy minerals. Without the support of magnesium, vitamin D, and other important nutrients, calcium couldn't do its job. In this chapter, we've gone over a lot of supplements that help prevent osteoporosis. But don't worry about putting it all together. We'll do that for you in the final chapter of this book.

8

IPRIFLAVONE: THE NEW NUTRITIONAL MEDICINE

In the last seven chapters we've explored how your bones work and what can happen to them and to you when they don't. We've also talked about natural ways to help build and maintain healthy bone. Now we're ready to tell you about a new, natural substance that works as well as the most commonly used medications for osteoporosis—without any potential risk of increased cancer or other side effects. Sound too good to be true? It's not. This extraordinary substance is called **ipriflavone,** and it could well be the biggest breakthrough yet in osteoporosis prevention and treatment. In this chapter, we'll talk about what ipriflavone is, describe the research behind it, and outline how it can work for you as a safe, natural, and extraordinarily effective treatment for osteoporosis.

Nature's Answer to Estrogen

If you're a woman, it's likely that you have already had to—or soon will have to—grapple with the complex issue of treating osteoporosis with traditional drug regimens. As we've seen, the most common of these is estrogen replacement therapy (ERT). In spite of the controversy surrounding estrogen replacement therapy, one fact is clear: hormonal therapy *does* treat osteoporosis. But its potential for unwanted side effects—most notably, breast and uterine cancers—can be very frightening.

Recent research has identified natural substances that mimic the beneficial aspects of estrogens, without their potential side effects. The most promising of these substances are **isoflavones,** which we discussed in Chapter 6, and a significant amount of data has been published on their ability to maintain healthy bones.

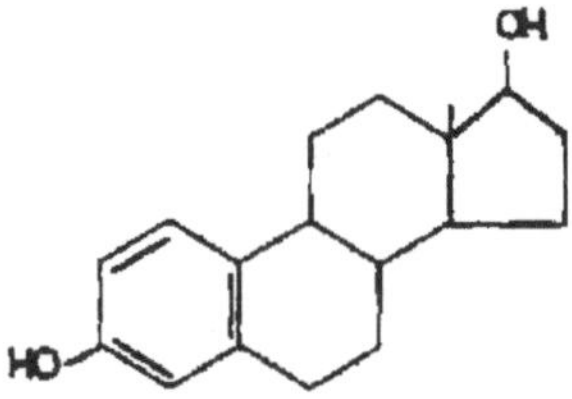

17β-Estradiol

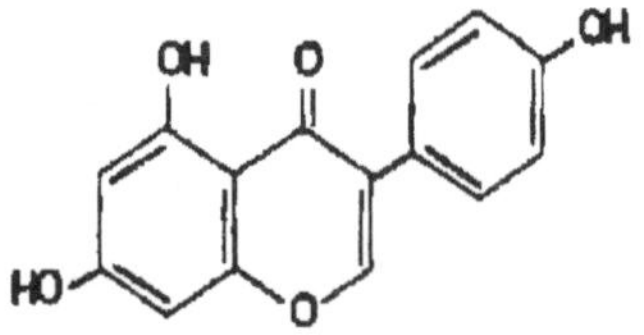

Genistein   Daidzein

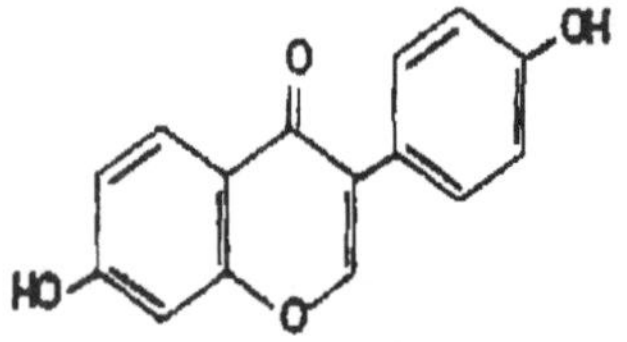

Figure 8-1. Comparative structures of isoflavones and estrogen.

Based on that work, researchers took isoflavones one step further and discovered how to refine and synthesize from them the compound known as ipriflavone. But before we talk about ipriflavone specifically, let's look at the action of isoflavones in general to understand how ipriflavone works.

Isoflavones: The Raw Form of Ipriflavone

Flavonoids are the most common compounds found in plants—including the fruits and vegetables we eat on a daily basis. Within the category of flavonoids are substances called isoflavones. **Isoflavones** are so-called plant estrogens that have positive influences on bone similar to the effects of estrogen. But while estrogen has been associated with an increased risk of cancer, plant estrogens can help *reduce* the risk of cancer. Chemically, isoflavones look very much like the estrogen produced by women. In the body, they're converted into very weak forms of estrogen that are only about 1/1000 as potent as the body's estrogen. (See Figure 8-1.)

In spite of their significantly weaker form, isoflavones still have powerful bone building effects. They do not, however, have the potential side effect of causing cancer. Because the body recognizes them as estrogen, isoflavones compete for receptor sites normally occupied by estrogen. Here's how it works. Every cell has a parking space (the receptor site) that's earmarked for certain compounds.

Now imagine the bloodstream as a highway and chemical compounds as cars. The chemical compounds "drive" through the bloodstream, looking for their designated parking spots. Because isoflavones look identical to estrogen, they can park in the same spot, forcing estrogen cells to keep circling the bloodstream block, looking for a parking place, or going to the liver and getting broken down.

While estrogen does indeed keep bones healthy, it also has the capability of promoting cell growth, which when unchecked develops into cancer. If estrogen can't park on a cell because isoflavone is parked there, it can't cause that kind of cell growth. And since isoflavone is such a weak form, it doesn't have the same effects on cells as estrogen does. The bottom line is that isoflavones work like estrogen to promote healthy bones, but do not have its deleterious side effects, especially the potential for cancer.

Now what's the connection between isoflavones and ipriflavone? In short, ipriflavone is a *derivative* of isoflavones and is organically synthesized from isoflavones. The term *synthesized* implies that ipriflavone doesn't exist in nature, which is partly true: ipriflavone has been identified only in trace amounts in *propolis* (a resinous material produced by bees) and in certain plants. For the most part, ipriflavone is produced as a supplement via the synthesis of isoflavones.

The History of Ipriflavone

Ipriflavone can safely increase bone mass and density without the deadly side effects of ERT and other traditional treatments. It's widely accepted around the world and is a registered drug for the treatment of osteoporosis in Europe, Japan, and Argentina. But like any rising star, ipriflavone had to start somewhere. In this case, it was in a Hungarian laboratory in the late 1960s, where it was used as a feed additive for veterinary applications. Animal studies over the next few years spurred scientists to further investigate this new compound. Some of the findings that piqued the interest of scientists showed that ipriflavone:

- Increases the total amount of calcium retained in bones.
- Preserves bone by inhibiting the activity of bone breaking osteoclasts.

- Promotes the production and activity of bone building osteo-blasts.
- Decreases the loss of minerals from bones that occurs when a person's diet is deficient in calcium and vitamin D.
- Decreases the activity of nitric oxide, which results in decreased activity of bone breaking osteoclasts.

One of the most interesting animal studies showed that high doses of ipriflavone increased the density of bone and its functional properties—that is, how well bone works to support the body and how resistant it is to fractures. This study was noteworthy for two reasons. First, the test subjects were males. (Most osteoporosis research has focused on females, but plenty of men also get osteoporosis.) Second, the function and strength properties of bone were improved without changing the ratio of minerals native to bone. These animal studies were convincing enough to pave the way for human studies with ipriflavone, which we'll look at in a moment. But first, let's see how ipriflavone helps treat osteoporosis.

Ipriflavone and Healthy Bones: How It Works

Like isoflavones, ipriflavone's chemical structure is similar to the chemical structure of estrogen. Consequently, the body uses it in much the same way to help reduce bone loss. As we've seen, estrogens inhibit the activity of osteoclasts, which break down bone, while enhancing the activity of osteoblasts, which build up bone. Research has shown that ipriflavone and its metabolites (see Figure 8-2) work in the same way:

- Ipriflavone may inhibit bone breakdown by activating ipriflavone receptors on the surface of osteoclast cells. These ipriflavone receptors have yet to be identified in human osteoclast cells.
- Ipriflavone also appears to enhance bone growth, both by boosting the activity of bone-building osteoblasts and by increasing the production of bone matrix proteins.
- Ipriflavone may promote the repair of fractures in long bones like those in the legs by transforming certain kinds of bone marrow cells into osteoblasts.
- Ipriflavone may enhance the secretion of calcitonin, the primary bone building hormone.
- Ipriflavone works primarily in bone tissue and not on other organs. Thus, it doesn't have the deleterious effects that estrogen does, like increased risk of uterine cancer.

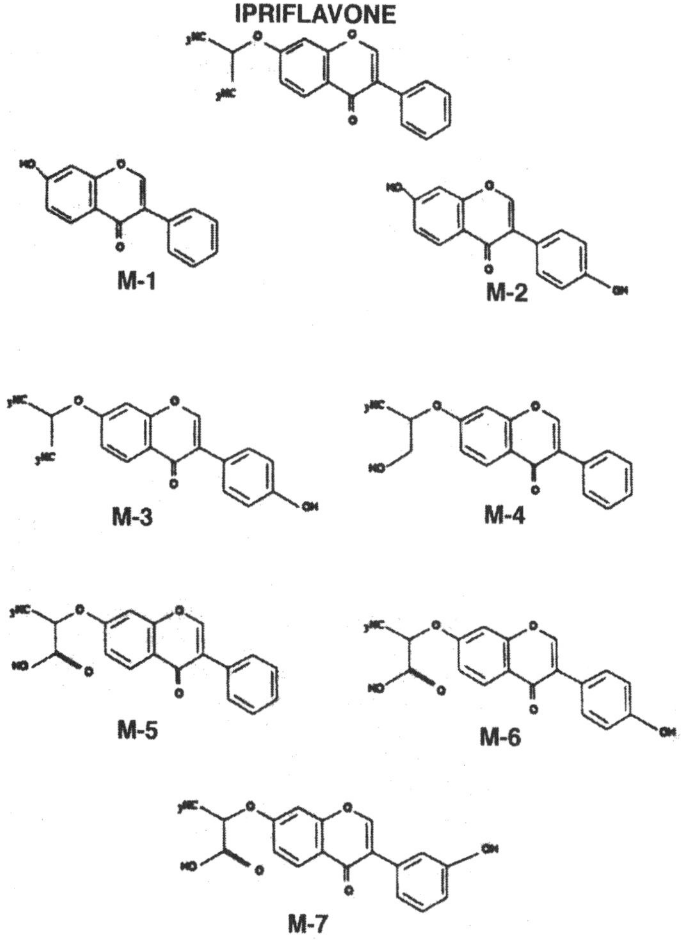

IPRIFLAVONE

Figure 8-2. Biological metabolites of ipriflavone.

Ipriflavone as a Complementary Therapy

As we've noted, isoflavones are recognized by the body as estrogen. Ipriflavone, on the other hand, isn't exactly *recognized* as estrogen but rather, *mimics* the action of estrogen—a slightly different mechanism with the same end result. So ipriflavone can work in the body like estrogen, without estrogen's negative effects.

With ERT, the lower the dose of estrogen, the lower the risk of side effects—but also, the lower the efficacy of the therapy. And at higher doses, the risk of cancer increases. This is where ipriflavone comes in as a complementary treatment to estrogen replacement therapy (ERT). In a study published in the prestigious *Osteoporosis*

International Journal, researchers found that ipriflavone, given along with very low doses of estrogen, increased bone mass—without the side effects associated with conventional ERT. So if you're a woman facing the prospect of ERT, you now have another alternative.

Ipriflavone can be a complementary therapy to other compounds as well. Combination therapies using ipriflavone and other bone building compounds like calcium may be more beneficial than ipriflavone used alone. The most impressive human studies on osteoporosis have used ipriflavone in conjunction with calcium, generally in the range of 500 mg to 1000 mg a day. Studies have also shown that ipriflavone, in conjunction with vitamin D, can help reduce postmenopausal bone loss better than either of these two substances alone.

Ipriflavone and Human Studies

Dozens of animal studies have proved that ipriflavone can protect bones without dangerous side effects. But we're not lab rats—our primary interest is in ipriflavone's application to our needs. And as far as human studies are concerned, the results are clear and remarkable: ipriflavone can prevent and treat osteoporosis without the side effects of conventional drug therapies. In addition, ipriflavone *not only helps prevent bone breakdown, it encourages bone formation,* so it's like putting money in the bone bank. Another positive point: ipriflavone actually decreases the acute and chronic pain associated with osteoporosis. Here are some of the more compelling results:

• Ipriflavone works better than prescription calcitonin in boosting bone mass. One study of postmenopausal women found that, compared to calcitonin, ipriflavone more than doubled bone mass density. Ipriflavone may even have the added effect of increasing calcitonin production in the body. This would be very valuable, because calcitonin is one of the hormones associated with bone building.

• Ipriflavone decreases bone loss and helps relieve pain associated with bone disorders in general. One study examined the effect of ipriflavone on Paget's disease, a disorder that results in significant bone loss and pain. People with Paget's were given either 600 mg or 1200 mg of ipriflavone a day. After one month, they showed a substantial reduction in bone loss—probably because of ipriflavone's ability to decrease the activity of osteoclasts. Another important point: the people in the study noted that their pain was significantly reduced after taking ipriflavone.

• Ipriflavone reduces bone breakdown. Another study looked at the effects of ipriflavone in men and women with hyperparathyroidism—a disease in which the body produces too much parathyroid hormone (PTH), one of the main hormones that promotes bone breakdown. The people in the study were given 600 mg a day of ipriflavone for up to forty-two days. All of them showed signs of reduced bone breakdown—probably because ipriflavone prevents PTH from indirectly activating osteoclast cells that break down bone.

• Ipriflavone works better than calcium for bone health. One small-scale study examined women who had recently undergone hysterectomies and who had subsequently experienced symptoms of menopause. Those who took 600 mg of ipriflavone, along with 500 mg of calcium every day showed decreased bone breakdown while maintaining the density of bone in the forearm—an indication of overall bone health. After one year, women who took calcium alone actually showed an *increased* rate of bone turnover and a 4.5 percent *decrease* in forearm bone density. In other words, calcium alone isn't the answer, and calcium tends to work better in the presence of ipriflavone.

• Ipriflavone increases bone density while slowing bone loss. A two-year study investigated the bone building effects of ipriflavone on the vertebrae. Nearly two hundred postmenopausal women with low spinal bone density took 1000 mg of calcium a day, along with either 200 mg of ipriflavone or an inactive placebo. After six months, the women who received the ipriflavone and calcium supplementation showed an increase in spinal bone density. The increase was clinically significant and indicative of a decreased risk of fracture. On the other hand, bone density in the women who received calcium and an inactive placebo showed an overall *decrease* after two years.

• Ipriflavone helps to prevent the loss of vertebral bone. Another two-year double-blind study examined the effect of ipriflavone on preventing postmenopausal spinal bone loss. One group of people received 600 mg of ipriflavone plus 1000 mg of calcium per day, while another group received only a placebo. The difference between the two groups was significant: women who took ipriflavone showed no decrease in vertebral bone loss.

These are dramatic findings. What they say is that ipriflavone can help prevent and treat osteoporosis better than prescription drugs, and that it has the added effect of decreasing pain—with no negative side effects.

The Good Side Effects

We've talked a lot about the deadly side effects of prescription drugs. In contrast, ipriflavone has some pretty wonderful side effects. Because it works in the body like estrogen, it has all the good qualities of estrogen. Ipriflavone helps to minimize hot flashes associated with menopause. Ipriflavone may also help prevent high blood cholesterol associated with estrogen deficiency, reduce bone pain, and even increase immunity.

Summary of Selected Human Ipriflavone Studies

Following is a summary of some of the most compelling studies regarding the safety and efficacy of ipriflavone. Show this to your doctor—it can help answer any questions he or she may have about ipriflavone and bone health.

Agnusdei, D., et al, *Calcified Tissue International*, 1997
This two-year, double-blind, placebo-controlled, multicenter study investigated the efficacy and long-term safety of ipriflavone. A total of 149 osteoporotic women was randomly divided into two groups. The first group was given 600 mg of ipriflavone plus 1000 mg of calcium each day. The second group was given a placebo. Those who received the ipriflavone plus calcium experienced a significant increase in bone mineral density and general mobility. They also experienced a reduction in bone pain and bone turnover, and were subject to fewer vertebral fractures than those taking the placebo. Overall, the study demonstrated the long-term safety of ipriflavone, its ability to increase bone density, and its possible application as a fracture preventative in patients with osteoporosis.

Gennari, C., et al, *Calcified Tissue International*, 1997
This two-year, double-blind, placebo-controlled multicenter study was conducted to evaluate the efficacy and tolerability of a daily regimen of 600 mg of ipriflavone plus 1000 mg calcium. A group of 453 postmenopausal women with low bone mass was divided into two groups, with one group receiving the ipriflavone plus calcium and the other receiving a placebo. Those who received ipriflavone-plus-calcium had a significant effect preventing bone loss effect, deceased bone turnover, and increased bone density

compared to the placebo group. Only minor gastrointestinal side effects were noted among both groups.

Adami, S., et al, *Osteoporosis International*, 1977.
This Two-year, double-blind, placebo-controlled study evaluated the efficacy of a daily dose of 600 mg of ipriflavone plus 1000 mg of calcium. A total of 250 postmenapausal women with low bone mineral density was divided into two groups, with one group receiving ipriflavone plus calcium and the other, a placebo. Complete blood work was monitored throughout treatment. Only minor gastrointestinal complaints were noted in both groups. The results indicated that the women in the ipriflavone-plus-calcium group maintained their bone mass density and experienced a decrease in bone turnover compared to the placebo group.

Agnusdei, D., et al, *Calcified Tissue International*, 1997
This two-year, double-blind, placebo-controlled, multicenter study evaluated the efficacy of a daily dose of 600 mg of ipriflavone and 1000 mg of calcium in post-menopausal women. A total of 198 postmenopausal women with low vertebral bone density was divided into two groups, with one group receiving ipriflavone plus calcium and the other receiving a placebo. A significant increase in vertebral bone density and decreased bone turnover was found in the ipriflavone-plus-calcium group. Routine blood, liver, and kidney function tests were performed before and after treatment. Only minor adverse reactions (mainly gastrointestinal complaints) occurred—and to a similar extent in both groups. The results demonstrated the safety of ipriflavone and how it can prevent bone loss in postmenopausal women with low bone mass.

De Aloysio, D., et al, *Gynecology & Endocrinology*, 1997
This one-year study evaluated the effects of either ipriflavone alone or ipriflavone plus low-dose hormone replacement therapy in the prevention of postmenopausal bone loss. The results demonstrated that ipriflavone and low-dose estrogen are effective in the prevention of postmenopausal osteopenia.

Agnusdei, D., et al, *Osteoporosis International*, 1995
This one-year, multicenter study evaluated the efficacy of 600 mg of ipriflavone and low-dose estrogen (0.30 mg/day) on bone loss in 83 early postmenopausal women. The adverse side effects of the ipriflavone plus estrogen were insignificant and were similar to those experienced by the women receiving the placebo. The results

suggest that the combination therapy produces a significant increase in bone density.

Ushiroyama, T., et al, *International Journal of Gynecology & Obstetrics*, **1995**
This study investigated the efficacy of a daily dose of 600 mg ipriflavone plus vitamin D in preventing postmenopausal bone loss. A total of 98 postmenopausal women was divided into three groups. The first group took ipriflavone plus vitamin D. The second group took ipriflavone only, while the third group took vitamin D only. The significant reduction in vertebral bone loss among those receiving the combination therapy suggests that this combination could prevent postmenopausal bone loss.

Zsuzanna, B., *Acta Pharmacology Hungary*, **1995**
This summary of the clinical results of ipriflavone as a nonhormonal, antiosteoporotic alternative to estrogen took note of ipriflavone's efficacy in decreasing acute and chronic back pain due to osteoporosis. It also noted that ipriflavone's rapid metabolization by the body caused it to be quickly eliminated before it could cause any long-term side effects.

Valente, M., et al, *Calcified Tissue International*, **1994**
This one-year, placebo-controlled, double-blind study evaluated the efficacy of 600 mg of ipriflavone plus 1000 mg of calcium on bone density in postmenopausal women with low bone mass. A total of 40 postmenopausal women was divided into two groups, with the first group receiving a daily dose of 600 mg of ipriflavone plus 1000 mg of calcium and the second group receiving a placebo. After one year, those receiving the ipriflavone plus calcium showed a significantly greater increase in bone mass density and a significantly lower bone turnover rate than those receiving the placebo.

Melis, G.B., et al, *Journal of Endocrinology Investigation*, **1992**
This study investigated the comparative estrogenic effects of ipriflavone and estrogen therapy in postmenopausal women. The results confirmed ipriflavone's inability to elicit estrogenic activity in other organs. This was important since ipriflavone shows the bone building properties of estrogen without the estrogenic effects on other organ systems.

Melis, G.B., et al, *Bone Mineralization*, **1992**
This one-year, double-blind, placebo-controlled study evaluated the impact of a daily dose of 600 mg of ipriflavone plus 1000 mg of

calcium on bone mineral loss in postmenopausal women. A total of 133 postmenopausal women was divided into three groups. The first group took ipriflavone plus calcium. The second group took estrogen only, and the third group took a placebo. After one year, the group taking ipriflavone plus a low dose of estrogen showed a significant increase in bone density in comparison with the other two groups. The results demonstrated that the addition of ipriflavone improves the effect of low-dose estrogen on postmenopausal symptoms.

Passeri, M., et al, *Bone Mineralization*, 1992
This one-year, double-blind, placebo-controlled study evaluated the efficacy of 600 mg of ipriflavone plus 1000 mg of calcium on bone mass in osteoporotic women. A total of 28 osteoporotic women was divided into two groups, with one group taking ipriflavone plus calcium, and the other taking a placebo. After one year, a significant increase in bone mineral density and a decrease in bone turnover was noted in the ipriflavone-plus-calcium group.

Nakamura, S., et al, *Calcified Tissue International*, 1992
This study evaluated the effects of administering a daily dose of 600 mg of ipriflavone to elderly female subjects after rapid calcium infusion. The results indicated that ipriflavone inhibits bone loss by speeding the secretion of calcitonin.

The Safety of Ipriflavone

We've seen that ipriflavone has dramatic effects on osteoporosis. And here's the best part: in numerous studies, ipriflavone showed no significant side effects. A major paper rounded up the data on safety and efficacy of ipriflavone, in sixty clinical studies performed in Italy, Japan, and Hungary and involving more than 2769 people. The paper looked at long-term (two-year) reactions to ipriflavone and found *no significant side effects* from its use.

The few side effects that were noted were mainly gastrointestinal in nature. It's possible that these effects were caused by the calcium used in conjunction with ipriflavone in the studies, rather than by the ipriflavone itself. The complaints that were noted, like bloating and constipation, are common and well-recognized side effects of calcium supplementation. As for the overall safety rating of ipriflavone therapy, no effects on the organs or other body systems have been seen, nor have there been any modifications of structural aspects of the bone.

While studies clearly support the safety of ipriflavone, one effect must be noted: ipriflavone has been reported to slightly and briefly raise liver enzymes, and may have an effect on the body's ability to metabolize certain drugs. The effect is similar to that of niacin, which is commonly used to reduce cholesterol and may also raise liver enzymes temporarily. If you're on other medications and you're taking ipriflavone, you should ask your doctor to monitor your blood work on a regular basis. You should also seek out a well-trained, nutritionally oriented physician to guide you in your treatment plan. The truth is that with or without ipriflavone, it's very important to boost your liver function if you're taking prescription medications. A nutritionally oriented physician can help you find nutritional compounds that support your liver and enhance its detoxification capabilities.

Liver Detoxification and Support

Following are several types of liver support compounds. The doses are set as minimums and may need to be adjusted at the direction of your health care practitioner.

- NAC (n-acetyl-l-cysteine): 500 mg
- Alpha Lipoic Acid: 200 mg
- Vitamin C (in buffered calcium ascorbate form): 500 mg
- Selenium (in yeast-free selenomethionine form): 100 mcg
- Standardized Turmeric: 200 mg
- Phosphatidylcholine: 500 mg
- Standardized Milk Thistle Extract: 200 mg
- Standardized Dandelion Extract: 200 mg
- Standardized Phyllanthus Extract: 200 mg
- Standardized Picrorhiza Extract: 200 mg

The long-term (that is, more than two years) effect of ipriflavone on bone density and bone mass, as well as possible side effects, are still being determined. A couple of well-designed studies have shown that ipriflavone is safe and effective over a two-year period. The benchmark of any effective treatment for osteoporosis is a reduction in the incidence of fractures. Ipriflavone has been shown to decrease the indicence of fracture, and long-term additional studies are under way. A three-year, multicenter trial measuring bone mass and density, the incidence of spinal and peripheral fractures, and side effects is now in process. This and many other long-term studies will continue to validate the safety and effectiveness of ipriflavone.

What It All Means

Ipriflavone seems to be the best bet yet for preventing and treating osteoporosis. Estrogen and other drugs may be effective, but who wants to take on the risk of cancer and other serious side effects? Ipriflavone is a safe and effective alternative to prescription drugs. Used in conjunction with diet, exercise, lifestyle changes, and other supplements, ipriflavone is one of the most important elements in a comprehensive prevention and treatment plan for osteoporosis.

Recommended resources for Ipriflavone: See Resource Section for a list of companies that sell Ipriflavone.

9

EXERCISING FOR HEALTHY BONES

Having read this far, you understand that osteoporosis is a lifestyle issue. Certain dietary changes, supplements, and new nutrients can help prevent and treat osteoporosis. But don't think you're going to get off that easy. For optimal bone health, you do have to start a regular exercise routine. The prevention of osteoporosis and its related fractures should focus on preserving and enhancing bone mass, preventing falls, and increasing muscle mass surrounding bone to provide cushioning and strength. A regular exercise routine can accomplish all of this and boost overall health as well.

What's Your Risk?

Are you at a higher risk for developing osteoporosis? The more questions you answer "yes" to, the higher your relative risk.

- Do you have a small, thin frame, or are you Caucasian or Asian?
- Has a female member of your family experienced bone fractures as an adult?
- Are you postmenopausal?
- Have you taken high doses of glucocorticoid drugs, or have you been on thyroid or heparin therapy for long periods of time?
- Do you eat more refined or processed foods (like pizza, white bread, and packaged snacks) than whole foods (like fruits, vegetables, whole grains, and beans)?
- Is your diet low in dairy?

•Is your diet very high in protein?
•Are you physically inactive?
•Do you smoke?
•Do you drink alcohol, coffee, and/or cola drinks in excess?

Bones are maintained in part by the forces applied to them. As we saw in previous chapters, the astronaut floating around in space will experience a decline in bone mass because her bones are not forced to rebuild in response to the forces of gravity and body weight. Along with the forces of nature, physical activity helps build stronger bones by stimulating them to adapt and become stronger. Jogging is a good example: when you run, the impact of your foot against the grass or track "shocks" your body into building stronger bones. In addition, the repetitious contraction of muscles and tendons during running or other exercise forces the bones to adapt to the new shape of the muscle. Our bones would soon break if the muscles attached to them became stronger and the bones themselves did not.

As we get older, strength and overall fitness decline, and we usually become less active. The result is not only a decline in general health but also a decrease in bone mass. This is not to say that decreased bone mass is inevitable: bone health, as well as strength and overall fitness, can be improved at any age with a carefully planned exercise program. Not only does exercise protect against bone loss, it may even *increase* bone mass in all age groups. Here are a few findings from the ever-growing body of research that relates physical activity to bone health:

• Regular exercise preserves bone mass and decreases the back pain associated with osteoporotic fractures in postmenopausal women.
• Exercise increases bone mineral density, especially during strenuous and moderate exercise like jogging and fast walking.
• Adequate amounts of continuous weight-bearing or aerobic activity slows bone loss, maintains bone mineral density, and may even increase bone mass in young adulthood.
• Exercise influences weight-bearing bones—like the legs and spine, which hold the body up—and possibly also non-weight-bearing bones like the arms, provided there is sufficient calcium in the diet.
• Exercise can increase postmenopausal bone mass, although only modestly, and is more likely to provide a bone forming influence with optimum hormone levels and adequate nutrition.

- Bone loss resulting from cortisol medications may be slowed or reversed with exercise.
- Regular weight-bearing exercise seems especially effective in preserving or increasing bone mineral density in younger and older postmenopausal women.
- The effect of exercise on bone may be site-specific—that is, only those bones that are surrounded by exercised muscles will grow.

Besides the obvious advantage of increasing bone mass, exercise can also help prevent fractures by enhancing balance, increasing strength, and boosting coordination. Aging creates changes in both the muscular and nervous systems that cause an increase in sway and a decreased ability to quickly correct movements affecting the center of gravity. The result? A greater number of falls in the elderly. Falls are the leading cause of injury-related deaths and morbidity among the older population. It is estimated that 30 percent of people over the age of sixty-five sustain a fall, and about 50 percent of those falls result in multiple hip fractures.

The injury from falling—and, often from fear of falling again—makes many people less active. That inactivity leads to bone demineralization, which leads to a further increase in fracture risk. It's a vicious cycle that can be remedied with exercise. Weight-bearing exercise increases strength, coordination, and balance, so it decreases the risk of falls. Exercise is important not only to prevent falling and fractures, but also to speed recovery after an injury resulting from a fall. In other words, if you thought you could while away your golden years as a couch potato, think again.

Type of Exercise

In the realm of bone health, not all exercises are of equal value. Even though all exercise has some beneficial effects on bone mass, the most effective kind of exercise is still under debate. One reason the jury is still out on this is the difficulty of implementing an effective and standard study. Small sample groups, high dropout rates, poor compliance, and a variability in exercise practices among subjects are common. These inconsistency factors lead to inconsistent results—and a lot of question marks.

One area on which most experts agree is that exercise that involves either weight or resistance is the most bone-beneficial. **Weight-bearing activity** is a term used to describe work performed against the force of gravity, like walking, jogging, hiking, tennis, and climbing stairs. **Resistance training,** on the other hand, involves the use of weights, such as barbells or Nautilus equipment, and is characterized by resisting, lifting, or lowering weights. Both are good; no one is sure which is better.

Weight-bearing exercise may be more likely to increase skeletal mass because of its role in stressing the bones through both gravitational force and muscular contraction. This dual action places the bone at an above-average stress level and stimulates it to adapt. Resistance training puts only muscular stress on the bones, and its benefits may not be as great as when implementing weight-bearing exercises.

Others contend that resistance training enhances bone mineralization and that its effects in preventing osteoporosis are equal to or greater than the effects of weight-bearing exercise. Resistance training does have its place in a well-rounded exercise program and may be more appropriate in cases of severe osteoporosis, where the risk of falling or fracture from impact is great.

Intensity and Duration of Exercise

Another area of debate centers on the importance of intensity versus duration. The level of effort you exert when you're lifting weights may be more important than how long you lift. Bone mass can be significantly increased by a strength regimen that uses high loads in short spurts, rather than prolonged and repetitive exercise. For example, lifting ten-pound weights for two minutes might be better for your bones than lifting five-pound weights for seven minutes. One study proved this point: when bone densities of power athletes (sprinters, jumpers, and hurdlers) were compared with bone densities of endurance athletes (middle/long-distance runners), power athletes had higher bone mineral densities in the spine than endurance athletes.

Whatever its form, all types of weight-bearing or aerobic training are correlated with bone density. The one that suits you best depends on your medical condition, level of physical fitness, and health care practitioner's advice. Another important point: incorporating a variety of exercise regimens may yield a synergistic effect greater than using any single one exclusively. We'll discuss this in depth a little later.

How Exercise Helps Bone

The biological mechanisms by which exercise benefits bone are not completely understood, but there are a number of possible factors. Exercise may increase blood flow to the bones, delivering vital bone building nutrients or creating small electrical currents called piezoelectricity, which stimulates bone growth. Physical activity may also affect the body's hormonal control of bone remodeling, somehow shifting it to the bone-formation mode. This second factor is a little more complex than it appears, and contains some seeming contradictions.

To understand the effect of exercise on hormones that affect bone health, let's revisit two substances associated with bone formation and breakdown—osteocalcin and parathyroid hormone (PTH). Investigators have found that, depending on the type of exercise, these two markers of bone metabolism fluctuate to varying degrees. **Osteocalcin,** a protein produced by osteoblasts that's involved in bone formation, has been shown to decrease in long-distance runners but increase during high-intensity training. Oddly enough, exercise also stimulates PTH secretion, which is associated with bone breakdown—a seeming paradox. We do know, however, that exercise benefits bone, and further research may be able to explain exactly how.

We also know that bone remodeling in response to exercise is a mechanical adaptation that regulates the strain placed on bone from two sources: the contraction of muscles and gravity. Bone responds to exercise because the strain placed on it is beyond what the bone is accustomed to. This is the same effect that body builders experience: they progressively lift heavier and heavier weights to build bigger and stronger muscles. Their subsequent larger muscles are their bodies' way of adapting to the ever-increasing stress of weight lifting. The bones respond in the same way, growing and becoming stronger in response to exercise.

The Best Exercises for You

Exercise is only as effective your own dedication, and the best exercise is the one that you will do on a regular basis. If you loathe running but love tennis, you're more likely to grab your tennis racquet than don your jogging shoes—and you'll probably play tennis longer and harder than you would run. Shop around in the exercise area, and expect to try several activities before finding the one (or ones) that suit you best. Bone mass gained from exercise is quickly lost when you stop exercising, so consistency is crucial.

According to the National Osteoporosis Foundation in Washington DC, the following exercises are the most effective in combating osteoporosis:

• Walking
• Stair stepping
• Hiking
• Dancing
• Weight training
• Jogging
• Skiing (downhill and cross-country)
• Aerobics (low-impact)
• Treadmills

The design of your exercise program will depend in part upon the severity of your bone loss, the risk of fracture, your current level of fitness, your past level of activity, and your willingness to stick with it. An exercise routine is a highly personal process, and the most beneficial bone building exercises are those listed above. If individual needs—like current bone mass or risk of fracture—aren't taken into account, an exercise program not specifically designed by you and for you may be ineffective and could result in injury. In general:

• The exercise program for building and maintaining peak bone mass in children and adults should include a variety of activities. (See the list above.)
• For people with lower-than-normal bone densities at the spine or hip, low-to-moderate activities like stair stepping, cross-country skiing, or hiking are recommended, as long as there's no extreme risk of fracture.
• People with extremely low bone density (thus, an increased risk of fracture) should avoid impact activities and stick to exercise programs like water aerobics, walking in waist- or chest-deep water, swimming, or cycling on a stationary bike.

The Big Four Exercise Considerations

The basics of any exercise program should have the four following components:

1. **Frequency** Frequency determines how often a particular activity is performed. Ideally, you should exercise three to seven times

per week, starting out at three and building up. Don't try to do it all in one week—it won't work. Your muscles and heart need time to adapt and improve in strength. Space out your higher-intensity workout days, substituting a lower-intensity activity on the days in between. For example, if you're lifting weights or playing tennis on Monday, Wednesday, and Friday, devote the days in between to less intense activities.

2. **Duration** How long you perform your exercise program is important as well. Twenty minutes to an hour of continuous activity is the ideal. Again, work up slowly—start with twenty minutes and gradually increase the duration of your program. Progress by adding five minutes to your workout every six to eight workouts, but if this feels too intense, cut back on the time.

3. **Intensity** The amount of force or power expended during a workout is another consideration. Intensity is typically measured as a function of heart rate, with fifty-five to eighty-five percent of maximum heart rate considered an adequate target range (see the chart below to calculate your target heart rate). When you step up the intensity of your exercise, you'll naturally breathe harder. But if you find yourself out of breath to the point of having to stop, you've pushed yourself too far. Back off a little and pace yourself. As you progress, your ability to exercise harder will increase. As for how hard you should push yourself, use the conversation test: you should be able to carry on a normal conversation during exercise, without wheezing and panting.

4. **Variety** The key to a successful exercise program is variety. Doing the same routine over and over again leads to boredom and possible injury from overworking the same muscles. Diversify your regimen: for example, jogging two days a week, playing tennis once a week, and lifting weights twice a week is a more balanced program than running five days in a row. Also, since the jury is still out on which form of exercise is the best, you're covering your bases by including some of each.

Calculating a Target Heart Rate

•Determine your resting heart rate. While you're relaxed, count your pulse rate for 10 seconds and multiply this number by 6. This is your resting heart rate—use it as a point of reference. If your resting heart rate is relatively low, you may want to choose a higher target heart range.

• Determine your maximum heart rate. Subtract your age from the number 220. This is your maximum heart rate.
• Choose an appropriate target range. Generally 55 to 85 percent of your maximum heart rate is recommended. The higher the number, the more strenuous the workout.
• Calculate your target heart range. Use the following formula. Multiply your maximum heart rate by your chosen target range. For example, suppose a forty-year-old woman wants to achieve a 60 percent (.60) level of her maximum heart rate:

$$220 - 40 = 180 \text{ (\textbf{maximum heart rate})}$$
$$180 \times .60 = 108 \text{ (\textbf{target heart range})}$$

Getting Started

Before you start any kind of exercise program, consult your physician or health care practitioner if you have any kind of health condition. He or she will determine your risk of injury and help design a program that's best suited to your condition. If you're in any stage of osteoporosis, you should also know your risk of falling before you start an exercise program.

• **Getting dressed** Just as the right routine is necessary for the safest, most effective workout, proper exercise attire is equally important. A pair of well-cushioned shoes will prevent undue discomfort and injury, and nonskid soles will reduce calluses and the risk of falling when you're exercising. Choose shoes that are appropriate for your specific routine: running shoes for jogging, walking, and running; tennis shoes for tennis; dance shoes for dancing. Wear loose-fitting clothing, especially in warmer weather, to allow more freedom of movement and prevent overheating.
• **Warming up** Before you start exercising, take ten or fifteen minutes to warm up with stretching. The idea is to gradually increase your heart rate and the blood flow to your muscles and bones to prevent pulled muscles and strains. When you begin exercising, start slowly and gradually increase the workload. Pace yourself and you'll be able to exercise longer without discomfort or injury.
• **Listening to your body** Forget about the "No pain, no gain" rule—it's a myth. Pain is your body's way of telling you that something is wrong. If you start feeling any discomfort or pain during an exercise program, stop immediately. If pain continues

after exercising, apply ice packs as needed, and if the pain or swelling hasn't subsided in two days, consult your health care practitioner.

- **Staying hydrated** Drink plenty of liquids before, during, and after exercise to prevent dehydration and to replace lost fluids. You should be drinking a minimum of six eight-ounce glasses of water a day, and if you're stepping up your exercise program, you should also step up your fluid intake. Water is best, but if you're engaged in a particularly heavy exercise routine, sports drinks that contain electrolytes (potassium, sodium, calcium, and magnesium) and carbohydrates can help replace minerals lost during intense exercise and restore electrolyte balance.

- **Eating right** When, what, and how much you eat before and after exercise are important factors in maximizing your workout routine. Complex carbohydrates like whole grains and vegetables provide energy for your workout and keep your body from breaking down protein stores to use for energy. Eat lightly before exercising to prevent cramps, and wait at least two hours after a big meal to exercise.

- **Cooling down** When you've completed your routine, don't stop all at once. Decrease your activity slowly, and then cool down with gentle stretching to prevent muscle cramps and stiffness. Drink a big glass of water after you've finished exercising to keep your body hydrated.

Tips for Trouble-Free Weight Lifting

- Lift and lower weights slowly to minimize the risk of injury.
- Perform resistance exercise like lifting weights every third day rather than every day, to allow your body to recover.
- If you feel undue stiffness and soreness after lifting weights, decrease your weights and repetitions by 25 to 50 percent.
- Apply ice to sore areas of the body immediately after lifting weights.
- If you feel pain or are limping, stop your weight lifting program until you feel comfortable again. Again, if pain or swelling hasn't subsided in a couple of days, consult your health care practitioner.

Staying Active

Ideally, exercise should become an intrinsic part of your life. Everyone can find time to exercise, we're only talking about half an hour a few days a week. But if you're crunched for time for a few days, or just not in the mood for a day or two, you can still stay active. And even during your regular exercise regimen, you can still incorporate ways to add more activity to your life:

- Look for more opportunities to walk: stroll to the store and take a walk in the park with a friend after lunch.
- If you drive to work, park your car farther away from the office and walk the extra distance.
- Take the stairs instead of the elevator.
- Do light calisthenics while you're watching television.
- If you're doing errands around the house, set a pace and time yourself, then try to break your old record the next time you do that chore again.

These little additions can substantially increase your overall activity level and you probably won't even notice them. And even though exercise is sometimes hard (they don't call it "working" out for nothing), you should still be having fun. If you feel yourself getting into a slump, vary your program: take tennis lessons, or explore other places to walk and run. Enlist a friend to exercise with you. And if you need a little extra encouragement, join a health club; it's a great way to make friends and establish something to look forward to.

Eating and Exercising

- Eat two to four hours before exercising, and don't eat a big meal right before exercising.
- Choose a meal higher in complex carbohydrates before exercising. Skimp on fat and protein—they're harder and slower to digest—and drink plenty of fluids to stay hydrated.
- Drink plenty of fluids *during* your exercise program. Water is the best choice, but sports beverages can replace minerals lost during exercise.
- After exercising, drink lots of water to replace what you've lost during your routine.

What It All Means

Exercise has so many benefits—including the prevention of osteoporosis—that any amount is better then none. Physical activity keeps tendons, ligaments, and joints flexible, relieves stress and anxiety, and contributes to mental well-being. It increases energy and endurance, reduces the effects of aging, and helps maintain a healthy body weight by boosting metabolism. You've known for a long time that regular exercise can combat such illnesses as heart disease, high blood pressure, diabetes, and obesity. And now you can add osteoporosis to that list. So the next time you start to switch on your favorite cable show, put on your running shoes instead and take a brisk walk in the open air. The television will still be there when you get back.

10

PUTTING IT ALL TOGETHER:
THE OSTEOPOROSIS SOLUTION

Without a doubt, nutrition plays a critical role in the prevention and treatment of osteoporosis. Ensuring the adequacy of many nutrients besides calcium is fundamental to any program designed to keep bones healthy. We now know that adequate nutrition and exercise are crucial for the development and maintenance of optimal bone mass. Often, patients with osteoporosis are individuals with optimal dietary requirements. These requirements vary with age, prescribed medications, appetite, and the presence of other diseases, so it is essential that progressive nutritional advice be sought. As reported by researchers at the Osteoporosis Research Center at the Creighton University School of Medicine, nutritional intervention in osteoporotic patients with hip fractures has been effective in reducing medical costs and improving patient outcome. Intervention begins with an evaluation of the patient's health history and nutrient intake. With this as a basis, a nutritional care plan is then designed to improve the patient's quality of life and speed recovery.

The choice is yours, of course, but by working with a progressive nutritionist or nutritionally oriented physician you can create the best plan of action for *you*.

In the preceding chapters, we've gone over all the factors that influence bone health. Now let's put all these factors together in a plan that can help you prevent or treat osteoporosis naturally. The most important points to remember are listed below. Copy this list and post it in your kitchen or bedroom as a constant reminder.

1. Avoid excess protein. In general, most people need between 50 and 63 grams of protein a day.
2. Cut down on caffeine, especially if your calcium intake is low.
3. Reduce your intake of sugar.
4. Drink alcoholic beverages in moderation.
5. Stay active, and exercise regularly—about three to seven times a week.
6. Quit smoking.
7. Eat more soy products.
8. Increase your intake of calcium and other minerals.

Every year, millions of Americans develop osteoporosis. The best way to prevent osteoporosis and related fractures is to increase bone mass and density with nutritional intervention. There are no magic bullets, and the pharmacological approach isn't the answer. Ultimately, medicine and nutritional science must be united. And nutritional therapy must no longer be considered *alternative* treatments, but rather an integral part of the whole medical care plan. Simply put, the most effective program involves a variety of nutritional agents along with changes in diet and lifestyle.

The following plan provides for the most effective nutritional supplement program to address osteoporosis. The heart of the plan is ipriflavone. It occupies a place in the *Estrogen Replacement Formula* and in the *Bone Building Support Formula*. The additional formulas you'll find listed will address any other specific concerns that may accompany your condition. As with any nutritional program, you must proceed under the guidance of a health care practitioner—either a nutritionally oriented physician or a progressive nutritionist who can work with your physician. *Don't try to treat yourself without the proper guidance and medical follow-up.*

The Foundation: Nutritional Medicine

The following two formulas are the foundation of the osteoporosis solution. The Estrogen Replacement Formula is specifically designed to treat osteoporosis, and the Bone Building Support Formula is for both prevention and treatment (along with the dietary and lifestyle changes we've talked about throughout this book). The supplements in the following protocols are to be distributed throughout the day and taken with meals.

Estrogen Replacement Formula

- Ipriflavone: 600 mg (200 mg, three times daily)
- Isoflavones: 100 mg (from soy isoflavone concentrates)

Bone Building Support Formula

- Calcium (citrate or glycinate): 1000 mg (1500 mg if you're not taking ipriflavone)
- Magnesium (citrate or glycinate: 500 mg
- Vitamin D (cholecalciferol): 400 IU
- Vitamin K (phylloquinone): 150 mcg
- Boron (glycinate): 3 mg
- Zinc (glycinate, citrate or gluconate): 30 mg
- Copper (glycinate or lysinate: 3 mg
- Silicon (horsetail or red algae): 25 mg
- Vitamin C (buffered calcium ascorbate): 500 mg to 1000 mg

Additional Support Formulas

The following formulas will provide additional support, depending on your specific condition. Again, supplements should be distributed throughout the day and taken with meals. And don't worry—you don't have to buy dozens of different supplements. Most of these are available in combination formulas. Ask for them at your local health food store, or check the resource list in the back of this book.

Liver Detoxification and Support Formula

If you have elevated liver enzymes, the following liver support formulas are recommended in addition to the estrogen replacement formula. Your health care practitioner will determine the length of time you'll need to take them.

- NAC (n-acetyl-l-cysteine): 500 mg
- Alpha Lipoic Acid: 200 mg
- Vitamin C (buffered calcium ascorbate): 500 mg
- Selenium (yeast-free selenomethionine): 100 mcg
- Standardized Turmeric (Curcumin) Extract: 200 mg
- Phosphatidylcholine: 500 mg
- Standardized Milk Thistle Extract: 200 mg

- Standardized Dandelion Extract: 200 mg
- Standardized Phyllanthus Extract: 200 mg
- Standardized Picrorhiza Extract: 200 mg

Homocysteine Modulators

If you have elevated homocysteine or cholesterol levels, or if you have a history of atherosclerosis, the following should be added to your supplement plan:

- Vitamin B_6 (pyridoxine): 25 mg
- Vitamin B_{12} (cobalamin): 200 mcg
- Folic Acid (folacin): 400 mcg

Cytokine Modulators

If tests have shown that you have elevated inflammatory cytokines, or if you're experiencing inflammation and pain, add the following to your supplement plan:

- Vitamin D (cholecalciferol): 400 IU (may be eliminated if it's contained in your other supplements
- Vitamin E (alpha tocopherol): 400 IU
- Quercetin (dimorphandra or eucalyptus): 1000 mg
- Standardized Curcumin (turmeric) Extract: 1200 mg
- Standardized Boswellia Extract: 800 mg
- Pycnogenol® (patented pine bark extract): 400 mg
- Omega-3 Fatty Acids (fish oils or algae): 2000 mg

Dairy-Free Bone Building Recipes by Lisa Turner

Country Breakfast Scramble

SERVES 4 TO 6

1 pound firm low-fat tofu, frozen and *½ cup sliced button mushrooms*
thawed *¼ cup chopped fresh tarragon*
1 teaspoon turmeric *½ teaspoon sea salt*
1 tablespoon olive oil *½ teaspoon black pepper*
½ cup chopped red onion

1. Drain tofu well and crumble into a medium mixing bowl. Add turmeric and stir until well blended.

2. Heat oil in a medium skillet and sauté onion and mushrooms until onion is translucent. Stir in tarragon, salt, and black pepper.

3. Add tofu and sauté for 3 to 5 minutes. Serve hot.

Emerald Sea Salad

SERVES 4

2 cups dried wakame *1 tablespoon brown rice syrup*
1 cup dried arame *1 tablespoon tamari*
¼ cup rice vinegar *¼ cup sesame seeds*
2 tablespoons toasted sesame oil

1. Soak wakame in warm, filtered water until soft (about 5 minutes). Drain well and cut into strips, removing tough center stem.

2. Soak arame in warm, filtered water until soft (about 5 minutes). Drain well. Combine with wakame in a medium mixing bowl.

3. In a small mixing bowl, combine vinegar, sesame oil, rice syrup and tamari. Mix until well blended.

4. Add vinegar and sesame oil mixture to sea vegetables and toss to coat. Stir in sesame seeds and refrigerate. Serve chilled.

Open-Sesame Salad

SERVES 4

2 teaspoons brown rice vinegar
1 teaspoon toasted sesame oil
½ teaspoon turmeric
½ teaspoon salt
¼ teaspoon white pepper
¼ cup egg-free mayonnaise

1 pound low fat tofu, frozen, thawed
  and drained
¼ cup diced celery
¼ cup grated carrot
2 tablespoons minced red onion
¼ cup soaked and drained hijiki
¼ cup sesame seeds

1. Combine vinegar, sesame oil, turmeric, salt, pepper, and mayonnaise in a small bowl and mix well.

2. Crumble tofu into a medium mixing bowl. Add mayonnaise mixture and blend well. Stir in celery, carrots, onion, hijiki, and sesame seeds and mix until well blended.

3. Cover and refrigerate for several hours or overnight to let flavors blend. Serve at room temperature in a pita pocket with a handful of sprouts or on a bed of field greens.

Broccoli Cauliflower Bisque

SERVES 4 to 6

1 tablespoon olive oil
1 small yellow onion, chopped
2 cloves garlic. minced
¾ pound broccoli florets
½ pound cauliflower florets
½ teaspoon sea salt

1 teaspoon white pepper
3 cups vegetable stock
1 8-ounce package silken tofu
¼ cup dry sherry
Parsley for garnish

1. Heat oil in a large saucepan and sauté onion and garlic until golden.

2. Add broccoli, cauliflower, salt, and pepper, and sauté until broccoli is bright green. Stir in vegetable stock and simmer, covered, until broccoli and cauliflower are tender.

3. Purée broccoli mixture with tofu until very creamy. Return to pot, stir in sherry, and warm through. Garnish with sprigs of parsley.

Red Lentil Soup with Arame

SERVES 4 to 6

2 teaspoons olive oil	*4 cups vegetable stock*
1 medium onion, diced	*½ teaspoon black pepper*
1 clove garlic, minced	*1 cup red lentils*
3 carrots, chopped	*¼ cup tamari*
½ teaspoon sea salt	*½ cup lightly soaked arame, drained*
2 tablespoons each fresh thyme, basil,	*well*
sage, and rosemary	*¼ cup sake*

1. Heat oil in a large pot and sauté onion, garlic, carrots, and salt until onion is translucent.

2. Add herbs, stock, black pepper, and lentils and bring to a boil. Lower heat and simmer 30 minutes.

3. Add tamari and arame, and cook for 15 minutes longer. Stir in the sake and serve hot.

Walnut Sage Pâté

MAKES 3 CUPS

2 cups cooked lentils	*1 teaspoon white pepper*
½ pound silken low-fat tofu	*½ teaspoon sea salt*
1 tablespoon olive oil	*½ cup chopped walnuts*
½ cup fresh sage, chopped, with stems	
removed	

• Combine all ingredients in a blender and purée until very smooth.

• Serve as a spread on bread or crackers or as a dip with fresh vegetables.

Collard and Carrot Raita

SERVES 6 TO 8

½ pound collard greens, chopped
2 cups soy yogurt
½ cup shredded carrot
¼ cup raisins

½ teaspoon sea salt
½ teaspoon black pepper
1 teaspoon ground cumin

1. Lightly steam collard greens, just until bright green. Rinse under cold water to stop cooking.

2. Blend yogurt with carrot, raisins, salt, pepper, and cumin.

3. Stir in cooled collard greens. Chill thoroughly before serving.

Baked Kale with Parsnips and Carrots

SERVES 6 TO 8

1 tablespoon olive oil
1 medium red onion, diced
1 ½ cups diagonally sliced carrots
1 ½ cups diagonally sliced parsnips
½ teaspoon black pepper

3 cups fresh kale, chopped, with stems
* removed*
¼ cup water
2 tablespoons tamari

1. Preheat oven to 350°.

2. In a medium skillet, heat oil and sauté diced onion, carrots, parsnips, and pepper until carrots and parsnips are barely tender.

3. While carrots are cooking, lightly steam kale, just until bright green (3 to 5 minutes).

4. Stir greens into carrot mixture and turn into lightly oiled glass casserole.

5. Combine water and tamari, and pour over the top of casserole. Cover loosely with foil, and bake at 350°; for 15 minutes.

Red Potatoes and Greens

SERVES 4

1 cup diced red potatoes, with skins on
1 tablespoon olive oil
1 cup chopped portobello mushrooms
2 medium shallots, minced
2 cloves garlic, minced
½ teaspoon salt
½ teaspoon black pepper
1 pound mustard greens, torn into large pieces with stems removed
¼ cup water

1. Boil potatoes in a medium pot with a tight-fitting lid until just tender (about 7 to 10 minutes). Drain well and set aside.

2. While potatoes are boiling, heat oil in a medium skillet and sauté mushrooms, shallots, garlic, salt, and pepper until shallots are soft and mushrooms are tender.

3. Add greens to mushroom mixture and sauté briefly (about 1 minute). Add water and cooked potatoes, cover, and steam until greens are tender. Serve hot.

Southern Style Turnip Greens

SERVES 4

1 tablespoon safflower oil
1 small yellow onion, minced
½ teaspoon sea salt
½ teaspoon black pepper
½ cup water
2 cups diced turnips
1 pound turnip greens, torn into medium-size pieces, with stems removed
2 tablespoons red wine vinegar

1. Heat oil in a medium skillet and sauté minced onion, salt, and pepper until onion is translucent.

2. Add water and turnips, cover, and cook just until turnips are tender.

3. Add turnip greens and steam until greens are tender and turnips are soft. Stir in vinegar and serve hot.

Spicy Gingered Greens

SERVES 4 TO 6

1 tablespoon light sesame oil	*½ teaspoon cayenne pepper*
2 carrots, grated	*1 pound chard, torn into large*
¼ cup freshly grated ginger	*pieces, with stems removed*
2 teaspoons tamari	*1 pound mustard greens, torn into*
2 tablespoons honey	*large pieces, with stems removed*
1 tablespoon mellow white miso	*¼ cup sesame seeds*
1 tablespoon rice vinegar	*¼ cup water*

1. In a medium skillet, heat oil and sauté carrots and ginger until carrots are tender.

2. While carrots are cooking, in a small bowl combine tamari, honey, miso, vinegar and cayenne pepper, adding water as needed to form a smooth paste.

3. Add chard, mustard greens, and sesame seeds to pan with carrots and cook just until greens are wilted.

4. Add water and miso paste to vegetables, stirring well to coat all ingredients. Serve hot, or refrigerate until completely chilled and serve cold.

Broccoli with Shiitake Cream Sauce

SERVES 4

1 large head of broccoli, washed well	*¼ cup finely chopped yellow onion*
1 tablespoon olive oil	*1 tablespoon whole wheat flour*
2 cloves fresh garlic, crushed	*1 cup calcium-fortified soy milk*
½ cup finely chopped shiitake mush-	*½ teaspoon salt*
rooms	*½ teaspoon white pepper*

1. Cut lower stems off broccoli and set aside. Slice broccoli tops lengthwise. Peel lower stems and slice into ½-inch strips.

2. Steam broccoli until bright green and just tender (5 to 7 minutes).

3. While broccoli is cooking, heat olive oil in a medium saucepan. Sauté garlic, mushrooms and onion until mushrooms are soft.

4. Add flour to mushroom mixture, and stir to coat all ingredients. Cook on low heat for 1 minute, stirring constantly to prevent browning. Slowly add soy milk, salt, and pepper, cooking over low heat for 2 to 3 minutes longer or until sauce is thick and bubbly.

5. Remove broccoli from steamer and arrange on a serving platter. Drizzle with sauce and serve hot as a side dish.

Grilled Ginger Cutlets

SERVES 4 TO 6

1 pound firm low-fat tofu
½ cup tamari
¼ cup brown rice vinegar
2 tablespoons honey
2 tablespoons finely grated fresh ginger
2 tablespoons sesame seeds

1 teaspoon toasted sesame oil
1 bunch scallions, finely sliced
1 tablespoon arrowroot powder, dissolved in ¼ cup cold water
1 tablespoon olive oil

Garnish: Sliced scallions and sesame seeds

1. Slice tofu into cutlets about ¼ inch thick and layer in a casserole dish.

2. Combine tamari, vinegar, honey, ginger, sesame seeds, and toasted sesame oil in a small bowl. Pour marinade over tofu slices, and let cutlets marinate overnight in refrigerator.

3. Remove cutlets from casserole and pour remaining marinade into a small saucepan. Add scallions and arrowroot to marinade, and cook over medium-low heat until thickened.

4. Heat olive oil in a deep skillet, and add tofu cutlets one layer thick, turning them as they brown.

5. To serve, place cutlets on a large platter, and drizzle with hot marinade. Garnish with scallions and sesame seeds.

Tofu Young

SERVES 4 TO 6

1 pound firm low-fat tofu
½ cup whole wheat flour
½ cup calcium-fortified soy milk
1 cup bean sprouts
½ cup sliced water chestnuts
¼ cup finely chopped scallions

½ cup sliced shiitake mushrooms
¼ cup lightly soaked hijiki, drained well
2 tablespoons tamari
2 tablespoons olive oil
1 to 2 cups mushroom gravy

1. Purée tofu with flour and soy milk. Stir in bean sprouts, water chestnuts, scallions, mushrooms, hijiki, and tamari. Batter should be fairly stiff—add flour if needed.
2. Heat olive oil in a deep skillet. Drop batter in by spoonfuls to form 3-inch pancakes about ½ inch thick.
3. Cook pancakes until golden brown, turning carefully. Drain well on paper towels. Serve over brown rice with Savory Mushroom Sauce (see below).

Savory Mushroom Sauce

1 tablespoon olive oil
2 cups finely chopped button mush-rooms
1 small yellow onion, diced
½ teaspoon sea salt

1 teaspoon black pepper
1 tablespoons whole wheat flour
1 cup calcium-fortified soy milk
½ cup stock or water

1. Heat oil in a large saucepan. Add mushrooms, onion, and salt and sauté until mushrooms are soft.
2. Add flour and stir until mushrooms are coated. Cook over low heat for 1 to 2 minutes, stirring frequently.
3. Slowly stir in soy milk and stock. Cook for 3 to 5 minutes longer or until thick and bubbly.
4. Transfer the mixture to a blender and purée on high speed, leaving some mushroom pieces for texture.

Southwestern Tempeh with Cilantro Pepper Sauce

SERVES 4

2 medium red peppers
1 tablespoon olive oil
½ cup diced red onion
1 cup diced green pepper
1 teaspoon salt
½ teaspoon black pepper
½ teaspoon cumin
¼ teaspoon cayenne pepper, or to taste

½ cup diced tomato
1 cup corn kernels, fresh or frozen and thawed
2 packages crumbled soy tempeh
¼ cup coarsely chopped fresh cilantro

1. Preheat oven to 400°.

2. Place peppers on a baking sheet and roast at 400°; for 20 to 25 minutes, turning several times until evenly charred on all sides. Remove from oven and wrap in a damp towel to cool.

3. While peppers are roasting, heat olive oil in a large skillet. Sauté onion, green pepper, salt, black pepper, cumin, and cayenne until onion is translucent.

4. Stir in tomato, corn, and tempeh. Cook over medium heat, stirring frequently, until tempeh is heated through and vegetables are tender (about 7 to 10 minutes).

5. Cut cooled pepper into strips. Combine in blender or food processor with cilantro and purée until smooth.

6. Arrange tempeh mixture on serving platter. Drizzle with red pepper sauce and garnish with fresh cilantro. Serve hot.

Rainbow Grains Stir-Fry

SERVES 4 TO 6

1 pound firm low-fat tofu
2 tablespoons tamari or soy sauce
1 tablespoon olive oil
½ cup sliced red onion
2 cloves garlic
1 cup broccoli, chopped
4 carrots, sliced on the diagonal

1 small red pepper, diced
1 small yellow pepper, diced
2 cups cooked brown rice
2 tablespoons coarsely chopped fresh basil

Garnish: fresh basil

1. Cut tofu into 1-inch cubes. Arrange on a medium plate and sprinkle with tamari or soy sauce. Set aside.

2. Heat oil in a medium skillet. Sauté onion, garlic, broccoli, carrots, red pepper, and yellow pepper until broccoli is just tender (about 5 minutes).

3. Gently stir in tofu and cook until golden.

4. Stir in brown rice and basil and heat through. Place on individual plates, garnish with sprigs of fresh basil, and serve hot.

Super Berry Smoothie

SERVES 2

1 medium frozen banana, sliced
1 cup fresh or frozen berries

2 cups calcium-fortified soy milk

- To freeze bananas: peel bananas and place up to four in a plastic bag. Freeze for 10 hours or overnight. Separate gently and cut into slices.

- Combine bananas, berries, soy milk in a blender. Purée until smooth and serve immediately.

APPENDICES

Where To Obtain Ipriflavone

Companies That Sell Ipriflavone and Ipriflavone Containing Bone Formulas

Solgar Vitamin & Herbs
500 Willow Tree Road
Leonia, NJ 07605
Phone (201) 944-2311
Fax (201) 944-7351
Web Site: www.solgar.com

Advanced Nutritional Products
Rockville, MD 20850
Phone (301) 987-9000
Fax (301) 963-3886
Direct Mail Order Number (888) 436-7200

Schiff (Weider Nutrition)
2002 South 5070 West
Salt Lake City, UT 84104
Phone (801) 975-5000
Fax (801) 972-2552

Natrol
21411 Prairie Street
Chatsworth, CA 91311
Phone (818) 739-6000
Fax (818) 739-6001

Natural Balance
PO Box 8002
Castle Rock, CO 80104
Phone (303) 688-6633
Fax (303) 688-8719

Where To Obtain Soy Isoflavones and Soy Concentrates

Companies That Sell SoyLife® Soy Isoflavones and Soy Concentrates

Solgar Vitamin & Herbs
500 Willow Tree Road
Leonia, NJ 07605
Phone (201) 944-2311
Fax (201) 944-7351
Web Site: www.solgar.com

Carlson Laboratories, Inc.
15 West College Drive
Arlington Heights, IL 60004
Phone (847) 255-1600
Fax (847) 255-1605

Schiff (Weider Nutrition)
2002 South 5070 West
Salt Lake City, UT 84104
Phone (801) 975-5000
Fax (801) 972-2552

Solaray, Inc.
1104 Country Hill Drive, #412
Ogden, UT 84403
Phone (801) 626-4956
Fax (801) 393-8215

Raw Material Sources For Ipriflavone
Soy Isoflavones (SoyLife®) and Pycnogenol®

For the source of Ipriflavone

Technical Sourcing International (TSI), Inc.
201 West Main Street, Suite 101
Missoula, MT 59802
Phone (406) 549-9123
Fax (406) 549-6139
Suppliers of Ostivone™—a special trademarked form of Ipriflavone

Nutratech
10 Washington Avenue, Suite 78-1D
Fairfield, NJ 07004
Phone (973) 882-7773
Fax (973) 882-9666

Chemtech
218 Rockaway Turnpike, Suite 692
Cedarhurst, NY 11516
Phone (516) 489-9365
Fax (516) 489-9372

Raw Material Sources For Soy Isoflavones (SoyLife®)

For the source of SoyLife®—special trademarked soy isoflavones and soy concentrates

Schouten USA, Inc.
3300 Edinborough Way
Minneapolis, MN 55435
Phone (612) 920-7700
Fax (612) 920-7704
Web Site: www.soylife.com
Contact: Laurent Leduc

Raw Material Sources For Pycnogenol®

For the source of Pycnogenol®—a special patented pine bark extract

Henkel Corporation
5325 South 9th
LaGrange, IL 60525
Phone (708) 579-6150
Fax (708) 579-6152

Osteoporosis Information Sources

The following organizations may be helpful in providing information about osteoporosis. Keep in mind that while ipriflavone has been extensively prescribed for treating osteoporosis in Europe, these organizations may not yet be aware of its impressive success rate, nor of the more than fifty human clinical studies demonstrating its safety and effectiveness.

American College of Rheumatology
60 Executive Park South, Suite 150
Atlanta, GA 30329
(404) 633-3777
Web Site:
    http://www.rheumatology.org/

Foundation for Osteoporosis
Research and Education
3120 Webster Street
Oakland, CA 94609
(888) 266-3015
(510) 832-2663
Web Site: www.FORE.org

Missouri Osteoporosis Foundation
Web Site: www.moof.org

National Institute of Health
9000 Rockville Pike
Bethesda, MD 20892
(301) 496-4000
Web Site: www.nih.gov

National Institute on Aging
P.O. Box 8057
Gaithersburg, MD 20898-8057
(301) 496-1752

National Osteoporosis Foundation
1150 17th Street NW, Suite 500
Washington, DC 20036
(800) 223-9994

National Women's Health Network
514 10th Street NW, Suite 400
Washington, DC 20024
(202) 628-7814

North American Menopausal Society
P.O. Box 94527
Cleveland, OH 44101-4527
(216) 844-8708
Fax: (216) 844-8708

Oasis Institute
7710 Carondelet
Clayton, MO 63105
(314) 862-2933

Osteoporosis and Related Bone Diseases
National Resource Center
1150 17th Street NW, Suite 500
Washington, DC 20036
(202) 223-0344
(800) 625-BONE
E-mail: orbdnrc@nof.org

Sacred Heart Osteoporosis Center
5151 North Ninth Avenue
Pensacola, FL 32504
(850) 416-6450

U.S. National Library of Medicine
8600 Rockville Pike
Bethesda, MD 20894
(800) 272-4787
(301) 496-6308

Nutritional Information Sources

Herb Research Foundation
1007 Pearl Street, Suite 200
Boulder, CO 80302-5124
(303) 449-7849

American Botanical Council
P.O. Box 201660
Austin, TX 78720-1660
(512) 331-1924

Council for Responsible Nutrition (CRN)
1300 19th Street NW, Suite 310
Washington, DC 20036-1609
(202) 872-1488

ANKH: Perspectives in Health and Well-Being
P.O. Box 236
Sayreville, NJ 08872
(908) 486-8984

Medical Nutrition Organizations

American Association of Naturopathic Physicians
2366 Eastlake Avenue, Suite 322
Seattle, WA 98102
(206) 323-7610

American Holistic Medical Association
4101 Lake Boone Trail, Suite 201
Raleigh, NC 27607
(919) 787-5146

American College of Alternative Medicine
P.O. Box 3427
Laguna Hills, CA 92654
(800) 532-3688

American Preventive Medical Association
P.O. Box 2111
Tacoma, WA 98401
(206) 926-0551
Fax: (303) 417-9378

Soyfood Information Sources

American Soybean Association
540 Maryville Centre Drive, Suite 390
P.O. Box 419200
St. Louis, MO 63141-9200
(800) TALK SOY

Soyatech Inc.
318 Main Street
P.O. Box 84
Bar Harbor, ME 04609
(207) 288-4969

Soyfood Center
P.O. Box 234
Lafayette, CA 94549-0234
(510) 283-2991

Soyfoods Association of America
1 Sutter Street, Suite 300
San Francisco, CA 94104
(415) 939-9697

United Soybean Board
16305 Swingley Ridge Drive, Suite 110
Chesterfield, MO 63017
(314) 530-1777

U.S. Soyfoods Directory
Indiana Soybean Board
423 West South Street
Lebanon, IN 46052-2461
(765) 482-4376

Exercise Information Resources

American College of Sports Medicine
P.O. Box 1440
Indianapolis, IN 46206-1440
(317) 637-9200
Fax: (317) 634-7817

American Council on Exercise
5820 Oberlin Drive, Suite 102
San Diego, CA 92121-3787
(619) 535-8227
Fax: (619) 535-1778

American Society of Exercise Physiologists
Tommy Boone, Ph.D., MPH
The College of St. Scholastica
ASEP National Office
1200 Kenwood Avenue
Duluth, MN 55811

Fifty-Plus Fitness Association
P.O. Box D
Stanford, CA 94309
(650) 323-6160
Fax: (650) 323-6119
E-mail: fitness@ix.netcom.com

GLOSSARY

Autoimmune disease A disease produced when the body's normal tolerance of its own constituents disappears, resulting in the attack and destruction of the body's normal cells by the immune system.

Bone density The volume of calcium and minerals within the bone tissue.

Bone mass The total amount of bone tissue in the skeleton.

Calcitonin A hormone secreted by the thyroid gland that tends to decrease the amount of calcium in the blood.

Calcitriol The biologically active form of vitamin D.

Cartilage The translucent and elastic tissue that composes most of the skeletal system during the early years of growth and development and eventually converts to bone. Cartilage then becomes an important player in keeping bone flexible.

Collagen An insoluble protein fiber that is the primary constituent in connective tissue (skin and tendons) and bone.

Corticosteroids Any number of hormonal steroid substances secreted from the adrenal glands; corticosteroids permit many biochemical processes to proceed at optimal rates.

Cytokines Compounds involved in regulating the immune response.

Estrogen A hormone usually associated with promoting the development of female secondary sex characteristics, including breasts.

Glycoprotein A molecule that is composed of a protein molecule linked to a carbohydrate molecule.

Hard bone Also known as *compact cortical bone;* the dense outer covering of a bone that surrounds trabecular bone; the outside surface of bone.

Herniated disk A rupture or protrusion of the cushioning gelatinous mass at the center of the intervertebral disk between the lumbar vertebrae of the spine, causing pain in the affected side.

Homocysteine An amino acid produced during metabolism of another amino acid called *methionine.* Homocysteine is regarded as a risk factor for heart disease and is implicated in other disease conditions.

Homocystinuria An inherited disease caused by the absence of an enzyme essential to the metabolism of homocystine.

Hormone A chemical messenger within the body that is secreted by one type of cell and acts on another type of cell.

Hydroxyapatite The chief structural component of bone; composed primarily of calcium phosphate crystals.

Hyperthyroidism Excessive activity of the thyroid gland, resulting in increased metabolic rate, enlargement of the thyroid gland, rapid heart rate and high blood pressure.

Hypothyroidism Deficient activity of the thyroid gland, resulting in decreased metabolic rate and a general loss of energy or strength.

Interleukin Any of several compounds produced by cells of the immune system that function in the regulation of the immune system.

Isoflavone A natural plant chemical that exerts estrogenlike effects in the body.

Malabsorption The inability to adequately or efficiently absorb nutrients from the intestinal tract.

Modulate To alter the function or status of something in response to a stimulant.

Monocyte A large white blood cell involved in the first line of immune defense and in the inflammatory process.

Ossification The process of bone formation—usually, the process by which cartilage is converted to hard bone.

Osteoblast Cells that form bone.

Osteoclast Cells that break down bone.

Osteocyte A cell that resides within special regions of adult bone and is involved in the maintenance of that bone.

Osteogenesis The formation of bone in connective tissue or cartilage (*osteo* meaning "bone" and *genesis* meaning "to begin").

Osteomalacia Also known as *"adult rickets."* A softening of the bones as a result of a deficiency of vitamin D.

Osteopenia A condition characterized by a decrease in bone density but not necessarily by an increase in fracture risk or incidence.

Osteoporosis A condition characterized by a decrease in bone mass as well as by decreased bone density and increased risk and/or incidence of fracture.

Parafollicular cells Found in the vicinity of or located around the cells of the thyroid.

Parathyroid hormone or **parathomone (PTH)** A hormone secreted by the parathyroid gland and associated with calcium utilization in the body.

Peak bone mass The maximum amount of bone one can achieve during skeletal growth.

Piezoelectricity Electricity or polarity that is a result of pressure, especially in crystals.

Prostaglandin A large group of biologically active compounds synthesized from unsaturated fatty acids. Prostaglandins have a wide assortment of biological effects, some of which are: fluid balance, blood flow, gastrointestinal function, and neurotransmission.

Proteoglycans Molecules found in the extracellular matrix of connective tissue that is composed of many carbohydrates linked to a protein.

Receptor A cell component that combines with a drug, hormone, or chemical to alter the function of that cell.

Remodeling The process of replacing old bone with new bone through the action of osteoclasts and osteoblasts.

Resorption The breakdown and assimilation of bone through the action of osteoclasts.

Skeletal system The rigid, supportive, and protective structure or framework of an organism; the bony or cartilaginous framework supporting the soft tissues and protecting the internal organs.

Spongy bone Also known as *trabecular bone*. A latticelike structure of bony tissue that makes up the inner portion of bone.

Vertebrae Any one of the thirty-three bony segments of the spinal column.

REFERENCES

Chapter 1

Tortora GJ and Grabowski SR, *Principles of anatomy and physiology*, 7th Edition, New York: HarperCollins, 1993.

Holick MF, Jrane SM and Potts JT Jr, *Harrison's principles of internal medicine* 14th Edition, edited by Fauci AS, Braunwald E, Isselbaucher KJ, Milson JD, Martin JB, Kasper DL, Hauser SL and Longo DL, New York: McGraw-Hill, 1998.

Cohn RM and Roth KS, *Biochemistry and disease: bridging basic science and clinical practice*, Baltimore, MD: Williams & Wilkins, 1996.

Schastnyi SA, Shchukin SI, Roslyi IM, Zubenko VG, Beliaev KR, Semikin GI and Morozov AA, Mechanism of action of electromagnetic fields biologically adequate to man, Vetn Ross Akad Med Nauk 1996, (5):51–4.

Fukada E., Piezoelectricity of biopolymers, Biorheology 1995, 32(6):593–609.

University of Texas Southwestern Medical Center at Dallas, Estrogen plays a key role in normal bone growth in men, http://www.swmed.edu/news/bone.htm, 1997.

Chapter 2

Amento EP, Vitamin D and the immune system. Steroids 1987, Jan–Mar;49(1–3):55–72.

Barton BR, IL-6: insights into novel biological activities. Clin Immunol Immunopathol 1997, Oct;85(1):16–20.

Benvenuti S, et al, Binding and bioeffects of ipriflavone on a human preosteoclastic cell line. Biochem Biophys Res Commun 1994. Jun 30;201(3):1084–9.

Berdyshev, EV, et al, Influence of fatty acid ethanolamides and delta9-tetrahydracanabinol on cytokine and arachidonate release by mononuclear cells. Eur J Pharmacol 1997, Jul 9;330(2–3):231–40.

Blok WL, et al, Pro-inflammatory cytokines in healthy volunteers fed various doses of fish oil for 1 year. Eur J Clin Invest 1997 Dec;27 (12):1003–8.

Bouillon R, et al, Immune modulation by vitamin D analogs in the prevention of autoimmune disease. Verh K Acad Geneeskd Belg 1995;57(5):371–85.

Bulger, EM, et al, Enteral vitamin E supplementation inhibits the cytokine response to endotoxin. Arch Surg 1997 Dec;132(12):1337–41.

Chan, MM, Inhibition of tumor necrosis factor by curcumin, a phytochemical. Biochem pharmacol 1995, May 26;49(11):1551–6.

Chaudhary LR, et al, Regulation of interleukin-8 expression by interleukin-1beta, osteotropic hormones, and protein kinase inhibitors in normal human bone marrow stromal cells. J Biol Chem 1996, Jul 12;271 (28):16591–6.

Cotrozzi G, et al, Osteoporosis: the recent findings on its etiopathogenesis, diagnosis and therapy. Clin Ter 1994, Apr;144(4):355–65.

D'Ambrosio, D, et al, Inhibition of IL-12 production by 1,25 dihydroxyvitamin D3. J Clin Invets 1998, Jan 1;101(1):252–62.

Dean DD, et al, Interleukin-1 alpha and beta in growth plate cartilage are regulated by vitamin D metabolites in vivo. J Bone Miner Res 1997, Oct;12(10):1560–9.

Dewhirst FE, et al, Purification and partial sequence of human osteoclast-activating factor: identity with interleukin 1 beta. J Immunol 1985, Oct;(135(4):2562–8.

Evans DM, et al, Nitric oxide and bone. J Bone Miner Res 1996, Mar;11(3):300–5.

Flanagan AM, et al, The effect of interleukin-6 and soluble interleukin-6 receptor protein on the bone resorptive activity of human osteoclasts generated in vivo. J Pathol 1995, Jul;176(3):289–97.

Fujita T, et al, Cytokines and osteoporosis. Ann NY Acad Sci 1990;587–371–5.

Gruber HE, Bone and the immune system. Proc Soc Exp Biol Med 1991, Jul;197(3):219–25.

Joe, B, et al, Effect of curcumin and capsaicin on arachidonic acid metabolism and lysosomal enzyme secretion by rat peritoneal macrophages. Lipids 1997, Nov;32(11):1173–80.

Kanematsu M, et al, Interaction between nitric oxide synthase and cyclooxygenase pathways in osteoblastic MC3T3-E1 cells. J Bone Miner Res 1997, Nov;12(1):1789–96.

Katz MS, et al, Tumor necrosis factor and interleukin-1 inhibit parathyroid hormone-responsive adeylate cyclase in clonal osteoblast-like cells by down-regulating parathyroid hormone receptors. J Cell Physiol 1992, Oct;153(1):206–13.

Keeting PE, et al, Evidence for interleukin-1 beta production by cultured normal human osteoblast-like cells. J Bone Miner Res 1991, Aug;6(8):827–33.

Kim GS, et al, Involvement of different second messengers in parathyroid hormone and interleukin-1 induced interleukin-6 and interleukin-11 production in human bone marrow stromal cells. J Bone Miner Res 1977, Jun;12(6):896–902.

Koncz, S, et al, Ipriflavone metabolite-III inhibits LPS-induced nitric oxide release from RAW-264.7 cells, Acta Physiol Hung 1996, 84(3):223–8.

Lerner UH, et al, Comparison of human interleukin-1 beta and its 163–171 peptide in bone resorption and the immune response. Cytokine 1991, Mar;3(2):141–8.

MacIntyre I, et al, Osteoclastic inhibition: an action of nitric oxide not mediated by cyclic GMP. Proc Natl Acad Sci 1991. Apr 1;88(7):2936–40.

Meydani, SN, et al, Oral n-3 fatty acid supplementation suppresses cytokine production and lymphocyte proliferation: comparison between young and older women. J Nutr 1991, Apr;121(4):547–55.

Muller, K, et al, 1 alpha, 25-dihydroxyvitamin D3 and a novel vitamin D analogue MC 903 are potent inhibitors of human interleukin-1 in vitro. Immunol Lett 1988, Apr;17(4):361–5.

Natale VM, et al, Does the secretion of cytokines in the periphery reflect their role in bone metabolic diseases? Mech Aging Dev 1997, Mar;94 (1–3):17–23.

Oelzner P, et al, Inflammation and bone metabolism in rheumatoid arthritis. Med Klin 1997, Oct 15;92(10):607–14.

Packer, L, et al, Pycnogenol(r): effects on the redox antioxidant network and nitrogen monoxide (NO) metabolism. Annual Meeting of the Oxygen Club of California 1998.

Papadopoulos NG, et al, Correlation of interleukin-6 levels with bone density in postmenopausal women. Clin Rheumatol 1997, Mar;16 (2):162–5.

Papanicolaou DA, et al, The pathophysiologic roles of interleukin-6 in human disease. Ann Intern Med 1998, Jan 15;128(2):127–37.

Pumarino H., et al, Cytokines, growth factors and metabolic bone disease. Rev Med Chil 1996, Feb;124(2):248–57.

Rogers MJ, et al, Biphosphonates induce apoptosis in mouse macrophage-like cells in vitro by a nitric oxide-independent mechanism. J Bone Miner Res 1996, Oct;11(10):1482–91.

Rosen CJ, T lymphocyte surface antigen markers in osteoporosis. J Bone Miner Res 1990, Aug;5(8):851–5.

Safayhi, H, et al, Boswellic acids: novel, specific, nonredox inhibitors of 5-lipoxygenase. J Pharmacol Exp Ther 1992, Jun;261(3):1143–6.

Safayhi, H, et al, Mechanism of 5-lipoxygenase inhibition by acetyl-11-keto-beta boswellic acid. Mol Pharmacol 1995, Jun; 47(6):1212–6.

Sato M, et al, Quercetin, a bioflavonoid, inhibits the induction of interleukin 8 and monocyte chemoattractant protein-1 expression by tumor necrosis factor-alpha in cultured human synovial cells. J Rheumatol 1997, Sep;24(9):1680–4.

Simpson RJ, et al, Interleukin-6: structure-function relationships. Protein Sci 1997. May;6(5):929–59.

Stabel, JR, et al, Influence of vitamin D3 infusion and dietary calcium on secretion of interleukin 1, interleukin 6 and tumor necrosis factor in mice infected with mycobacterium paratuberculosis. Am J Vet Res 1996, Jun;57(6):825–9.

Stabel, JR, et al, Vitamin E effects on in vitro immunoglobin M and interleukin-1 beta production and transcription in dairy cattle. J Dairy Sci 1992, Aug;75(8):2190–8.

Strivastava, KC, et al, Curcumin, a major component of food spice turmeric, inhibits aggregation and alters eicosanoid metabolism in human blood platelets. Prostaglandins Leukot Essent Fatty Acids 1995, Apr;52(4):223–7.

Toborek, M, et al, Linoleic acid potentiates TNF mediated oxidative stress, disruption of calcium homeostasis and apoptosis of cultured vascular endothelial cells. J Lipid Res 1997 Oct;38(10):2155–67.

Tsutsumi N, et al, Effects of KCA-098 on bone metabolism:comparison with those of ipriflavone. Jpn J Pharmacol 1994, Aug;65(4):343–9.

Urist MR, et al, Osteoporosis: a bone morphogenic protein autoimmune disorder. Prog Clin Biol Res 1985;187:77–96.

Watrous DA, et al, The metabolism and immunology of bone. Semin Arthritis Rheum 1989, Aug;19(1):45–65.

Wimalawansa SJ, et al, Nitric oxide donor alleviates ovariectomy-induced bone loss. Bone 1996, Apr;18(4):301–4.

Zarrabeitia MT, et al, Cytokine production by peripheral blood cells in postmenopausal osteoporosis. Bone Miner Res 1991, Aug;14(2):161–7.

Zheng SX, et al, Increase in cytokine production by stimulated whole blood cells in postmenopausal osteoporosis. Maturitas 1997, Jan;26(1):63–71.

Xu, YX, et al, Curcumin, a compound with anti-inflammatory and antioxidant properties, down regulates chemokine expression in bone marrow stromal cells. Exp hematol 1997, May;25(5):413–22.

Xu, YX, et al, Curcumin inhibits IL-1 alpha and TNF-alpha induction of AP-1 and NF-kB DNA-binding activity in bone marrow stromal cells. Hematopathol Mol Hematol 1997–98;11(1):49–62.

Xu J, et al, Cytokine regulation of adult human osteoblast-like cell prostaglandin biosynthesis. J Cell Biochem 1997, Mar 15;64(4):618–31.

Xu LX, et al, Osteoclasts in normal and adjuvant arthritis bone tissues express the mRNA for both type I and II interleukin receptors. Lab Invest 1996, Nov;75(5):677–87.

Chapter 3

Aisenbrey J, Exercise in the Prevention and Management of Osteoporosis. Physical Therapy 1987; vol. 67.7, p. 1100–05.

Albright F, PH Smith, AM Richardson, Postmenopausal osteoporosis: its clinical features. JAMA, 1941; vol. 116, p. 2465–74.

Barrett-Connor E, T, Holbrook, Sex differences in osteoporosis in older adults with non-insulin dependent diabetes mellitus. Journal of the American Medical Association 1992; vol. 268; 3333–7.

Barrett-Connor E, et al, Coffee-associated osteoporosis offset by daily milk consumption. JAMA 1994;vol. 271.4, 280–3.

Baum HBA, et al, Effects of physiologic growth hormone therapy on bone density and body composition in patients with adult-onset growth hormone deficiency. Annals of Internal Medicine 1996;125:883–90.

Bikle DD, et al, Bone disease in alcohol abuse. Annals of Internal Medicine 1985;103:42–8.

Bonnick SL, Osteoporosis handbook (Dallas, Tx: Taylor, 1997).

Borenstein DG, et al, Low back pain medical diagnosis and comprehensive management (Philadelphia, PA: Saunders, 1995).

Brown SE, Better bones, better body (New Canaan, CT: Keats, 1996).

Chalmers J, and Ho K, Geographic variations in senile osteoporosis. Journal of Bone and Joint Surgery 1970; 52B:667–75.

Chapuy MC, et al, Vitamin D3 and calcium to prevent hip fractures in elderly women. New England Journal of Medicine 1992; 327:1637–42.

Chrischilles EA, et al, A Model of lifetime osteoporosis impact. Archives of Internal Medicine 1991;151:2026–32.

Cumming RG, et al, Calcium intake and fracture risk: results from the study of osteoporotic fractures. American Journal of Epidemiology 1997; 145:926–34.

Cumming, RG, Klineberg RJ, Case control study of risk factors for hip fractures in the elderly. American Journal of Epidemiology 1994; 139:493–503.

Cummings SR, et al, Risk factors for hip fracture in white women. Study of Osteoporotic Fractures Research Group. New England Journal of Medicine 1995;332:767.

Cummings SR, Black, DM Rubin, SM, Lifetime risks of hip, colles' or vertebral fracture and coronary heart disease among white menopausal women. Archives of Internal Medicine 1989;149:2445–8.

Cummings S, et al, Future of hip fractures in the United States: numbers, costs and potential effects of postmenopausal estrogen. Clinical Orthopaedics and Related Research 1990;252:163–5.

Cundy T, et al, Bone density in women receiving medroxyprogesterone acetate for contraception. BMJ 1991;303:13—6.

Dalsky GP, et al, Weight-bearing exercise training and lumbar bone mineral content in postmenopausal women. Annals of Internal Medicine 1988;1008:824–8.

Dawson-Hughes B, et al, Effect of vitamin D supplementation on wintertime and overall bone loss in healthy postmenopausal women. Annals of Internal Medicine 1991;115:505.

Dawson-Hughes B, et al, Controlled trial of the effect of calcium supplementation on bone density in postmenopausal women. New England Journal of Medicine 1990;323:878–83.

Drinkwater BL, et al, Bone mineral content of amenorrheic athletes. New England Journal of Medicine 1984;311:277–81.

Felson David T, et al, Effect of postmenopausal estrogen therapy on bone density in elderly women. New England Journal of Medicine 1993; 329.16:1141–6.

Finkelstein JS, et al, Parathyroid hormone for the prevention of bone loss induced by estrogen deficiency. New England Journal of Medicine 1994; 331:1618.

Frost H, Pathomechanics of osteoporosis. Clinical Orthopaedics 1985; 200:198–225.

Grady D, et al, Hormone therapy to prevent disease and prolong life in postmenopausal women. Annals of Internal Medicine 1992;117:1016.

Greenspan FS, et al, Basic and clinical endocrinology (Appleton and Lange, 1997).

Heaney RP, et al, Calcium nutrition and bone health in the elderly. American Journal of Clinical Nutrition 1982;36:986–1013.

Hernandez-Avila Mauricio, et al, Caffeine, moderate alcohol intake, and risk of fractures of the hip and forearm in middle-aged women. American Journal of Clinical Nutrition 1991;54:157–163.

Hindmarsh JJ, Estes EH, Falls in older persons. Archives of internal Medicine 1989;149:2217–22.

Holbrook TL, Barrett-Connor E, Wingard DL, Dietary calcium and risk of hip fractures: 14 year prospective population study. Lancet 1988; 2:1046–9.

Hopper JL, et al, Bone density of female twins discordant for tobacco use. New England Journal of Medicine 1994;330.6:387–92.

Jensen G, et al, Epidemiology of postmenopausal spinal and long bone fractures: a unifying approach to postmenopausal osteoporosis. Clinical Orthopaedics and Related Research 1982;166:75–81.

Johannsson G, Rosen T, Bosaeus I, Sjostrom L, Bengtsson B, Two years of growth hormone (GH) treatment increases bone mineral content and density in hypopituitary patients with adult onset GH deficiency. Journal of Clinical Endocrinology and Metabolism vol 81:2865–73.

Johnston CC, et al, Calcium supplementation and increases in bone mineral density in children. New England Journal of Medicine 1992; 327:82–7.

Johnston CC, Jr, Slemenda CW, Pathogenesis of osteoporosis. Bone 1995; 17:19S.

Kelepouris N, et al, Severe osteoporosis in men. Annals of Internal Medicine 1995;123:452.

Kiel DP, et al, Hip fracture and the use of estrogens in postmenopausal women. New England Journal of Medicine 1987;317:1169–74.

Kiel DP, et al, Smoking eliminates the protective effect of oral estrogens on the risk for hip fracture among women. Annals of Internal Medicine 1992;116:716–21.

Kreiger N, et al, Dietary factors and fracture in postmenopausal women: a case control study. International Journal of Epidemiology 1992; 21:953–8.

Leichter I, et al, Effect of age and sex on bone density, Bone Mineral Content and Cortical Index. Clinical Orthopaedic and Related Research 1981;156:232–9.

Lukert BP, Raisz LG, Glucocorticoid-induced osteoporosis. Rheumatology Dis Clinics of North America 1994;20:629.

MacMahon B, et al, Cigarette smoking and urinary estrogens. New England Journal of Medicine 1982;307:1062–5.

Mazanec DJ, Grisanti JM, Drug-induced osteoporosis. Cleveland Clinic Journal of Medicine 1989;56:297–303.

McKinlay SM, Bifano, NL, McKinlay, JB, Smoking and age at menopause in women. Annals of Internal Medicine 1985;102:350–6.

Meuleman J, Beliefs about osteoporosis: a critical appraisal. Archives of Internal Medicine 1987;147.4:762–5.

Michaelson K, et al, Effect of prefracture versus post-fracture dietary assessment on hip fracture risk estimates. International Journal of Epidemiology 1996;25:403–410.

National Academy of Science, Recommended daily allowances (Washington, D.C.: National Academy of Sciences, 1989).

Nelson M, et al, Effects of high-intensity strength training on multiple risk factors for osteoporotic fractures: a randomized controlled trial. JAMA 1994;272.24:1909–14.

Nevitt MC, Epidemiology of osteoporosis. Rheumatic Disease Clinics of North America 1994;20.3:535–59.

Nilsson BE, Westlin, NE, Bone density in athletes. Clinical Orthopaedic and Related Research 1971;77:179–182.

Nordin B, International patterns in osteoporosis. Clinical Orthopaedics 1966;45.

Nordin BEC, Heaney, RP, Calcium supplementation of the diet: justified by the present evidence. BMJ 1990;300:1056–60.

Pace JN, Miller JL, Rose,LJ, GnRH agonists: gonadorelin, leuprolide, and nafarelin. American Journal of Family Practice 1991;44:1777–82.

Parfitt AM, Bone remodeling and bone loss: understanding the pathophysiology of osteoporosis. Clinical Obstetrics and Gynecology 1987; 30.4:789–811.

Paul TL, et al, Long-term L-thyroxine therapy is associated with decreased hip bone density in premenopausal women. JAMA 1988;259:3137–41.

Phillips S, et al, Direct medical costs of osteoporosis for American women aged 45 and older, 1986. Bone 1988;9:271–9.

Ray W, et al, Psychotropic drug use and the risk of hip fracture. New England Journal of Medicine 1987;316:363–9.

Reid IRR, et al, Effect of calcium supplementation on bone loss in postmenopausal women. New England Journal of Medicine 1993;328.7:460–4.

Riggs B, Melton L, Involutional osteoporosis. New England Journal of Medicine 1986;26:1676–86.

Riggs BL, Melton LJ, 3d, Prevention and treatment of osteoporosis. New England Journal of Medicine 1992;327:620.

Sambrook, et al, Prevention of corticosteroid osteoporosis. New England Journal of Medicine 1993;328.24:1747–52.

Seeman E, et al, Reduced bone mass in daughters of women with osteoporosis. New England Journal of Medicine 1985;320:554–8.

Seeman E, et al, Risk factors for spinal osteoporosis in men. American Journal of Medicine 1983;75:977–83.

Shangold MM, Exercise in the menopausal woman. Obstetrics and Gynecology 1990;75:53S–8S.

Sinaki M, Role of exercise in preventing osteoporosis. Journal of Musculoskeletal Medicine 1992;67–83.

Slemenda C, et al, Predictors of bone mass in perimenopausal women. Annals of Internal Medicine 1990;112.2:96–101.

Slovik DM, et al, Deficient production of 1,25 dihydroxyvitamin D in elderly osteoporotic patients. New England Journal of Medicine 1981; 305:372–4.

Sowers M, Epidemiology of calcium and vitamin D in bone loss. Journal of Nutrition 1993;123:413.

Spector TD, et al, Relationship between sex steroids and bone mineral content in women soon after menopause. Clinical Endocrinology 1991;34.1:37–41.

Stall GM, et al, Accelerated bone loss in hypothyroid patients overtreated with 1-thyroxine. Annals of Internal Medicine 1990;113:265–269.

Stampfer M, et al, Postmenopausal estrogen therapy and cardiovascular disease: ten-year follow-up from the nurses study. New England Journal of Medicine 1991;325.11:756–761.

Toh SH, Claunch BC, Brown PH, Effect of hyperthyroidism and its treatment on bone mineral content. Archives of Internal Medicine 1985;145:883–6.

Chapters 4 and 5

Adami S, et al, Bisphosphonate therapy of reflex sympathetic dystrophy syndrome. Annals of Rheumatic Disease 1997;56:201–4.

Aisenbrey J, Exercise in the prevention and management of osteoporosis. Physical Therapy 1987;67.7:1100–05.

Albright F, Smith PH, Richardson AM, Postmenopausal osteoporosis: its clinical features. JAMA 1941;116:2465–74

Bauer DC, et al, Broadband ultrasound attenuation predicts fractures strongly and independently of densitometry in older women. Archives of Internal Medicine 1997;157:629–34.

Bergkvist L, et al, Risk of breast cancer after estrogen and estrogen-progestin replacement. New England Journal of Medicine 1989; 321.5:293–7.

Bjarnason NH, et al, Tibolone: influence on markers of cardiovascular disease. Journal of Clinical Endocrinology and Metabolism 1997; 82:1752–6.

Bonnick SL, Osteoporosis Handbook (Dallas, TX: Taylor, 1997).

Borenstein DG, et al, Low back pain medical diagnosis and comprehensive management (Philadelphia, PA: Saunders, 1995).

Bowman BM, Miller SC, Elevated progesterone during pseudopregnancy may prevent bone loss associated with low estrogen. Journal of Bone Mineral Research 1996 Jan; 15–21.

Brandi ML, Flavanoids: biochemical effects and therapeutic applications. Bone and Mineral 1992;19:S3–S14.

Brown SE, Better bones, better body (New Caan,CT: Keats, 1996).

Carmel R, et al, Cobalamin and osteoblast-specific proteins. New England Journal of Medicine 1988;319:70–5.

Carter MD, et al, Bone mineral content at three sites in normal perimenopausal women. Clinical Orthopaedics 1991;266:295–300.

Cauley J, et al, Estrogen replacement therapy and fractures in older women. Annals of Internal Medicine 1995;122.1:9–17.

Chapuy MC, et al, Vitamin D3 and calcium to prevent hip fractures in elderly women. New England Journal of Medicine 1992;327:1637–42.

Christiansen C, Christiansen MS, Transbol I, Bone mass in postmenopausal women after withdrawal of oestrogen/gestagen replacement therapy. Lancet 1981;1:459–61.

Colditz Graham, et al, Use of estrogens and progestins and the risk of breast cancer in postmenopausal women. New England Journal of Medicine 1995;332.24:1589–93.

Cosman F, et al, Radiographic absorptiometry: a simple method for determination of bone mass. Osteoporosis International 1994;2:34–8.

Cummings SR, et al, Appendicular bone density and age predict hip fracture in women. JAMA 1990;263:665–707.

Cummings SR, et al, Bone density at various sites for prediction of hip fractures. Lancet 1993;341:72.

Cummings SR, Black D, Bone mass measurements and risk of fracture in caucasian women: a review of findings from prospective studies. American Journal of Medicine 1995;98:24S.

Cummings SR, et al, Risk factors for hip fracture in white women. Study of Osteoporotic Fractures Research Group. New England Journal of Medicine 1995;332:767.

Dalsky GP, et al, Weight-bearing exercise training and lumbar bone mineral content in postmenopausal women. Annals of Internal Medicine 1988;1008:824–8.

Dalsky G, Exercise: its effects on bone mineral content. Clinical Obstetrics and Gynecology 1987;30.4:820–32.

Dawson-Hughes B, et al, Effect of vitamin D supplementation on wintertime and overall bone loss in healthy postmenopausal women. Annals of Internal Medicine 1991;115:505.

De Groen PC, et al, Esophagitis associated with the use of alendronate. New England Journal of Medicine 1996;335:1016–21.

Designer estrogen builds stronger bones, USA Today, Dec 3, 1997.

Devogelaer JP, Clinical use of bisphosphonates. Current Opinions in Rheumatology 1996;8:384–391.

Dupont WD, Page DL, Menopausal estrogen replacement therapy and breast cancer. Archives of Internal Medicine 1991;151:67–72.

Ettinger BF, Genant HK, Cann CE, Long-term estrogen replacement therapy prevents bone loss and fractures. Annals of Internal Medicine 1985; 102:319–24.

Felson DT, et al, Effect of postmenopausal estrogen therapy on bone Density in elderly women. New England Journal of Medicine 1993; 329.16:1141–6.

Gallagher JC, Goldgar D, Treatment of postmenopausal osteoporosis with high doses of synthetic calcitriol. Annals of Internal Medicine 1990; 113:649–55.

Gardsell P, et al, Predicting various fragility fractures in women by forearm bone densitometry: a follow-up study. Calcification Tissue International 1993;52:348–53.

Genant K, et al, Osteoporosis: assessment by quantitative computed tomography. Orthopaedic Clinics of North America 1985;16.3:557–68.

Gorman C, Estrogen dilemma, Time 1997 vol. 150:23.

Grady D, et al, Hormone therapy to prevent disease and prolong life in postmenopausal women. Annals of Internal Medicine 1992;117:1016.

Grampp S, et al, Radiologic diagnosis of osteoporosis: current methods and perspectives. Radiology Clinics of North American 1993;31:1133.

Greenberg E, Breast cancer in women given diethylstilbestrol in pregnancy. New England Journal of Medicine 1984;311.22:1393–8.

Greenspan FS, et al, Basic and clinical endocrinology (Appleton and Lange, 1997).

Gregg EW, et al, Epidemiology of quantitative ultrasound: a review of the relationships with bone mass, osteoporosis and fracture risk. Osteoporosis International 1997;7:89–99.

Grey AB, et al, Effect of the antiestrogen tamoxifen on bone mineral density in normal late postmenopausal women. American Journal of Medicine 1995;99:636–41.

Grodstein F, et al, Postmenopausal hormone therapy and mortality. New England Journal of Medicine 1997;336:1769–75.

Guyton AC, Textbook of medical physiology (Philadelphia: Saunders, 1988).

Hans D, et al, Ultrasonographic heel measurements to predict hip fracture in elderly women: the EPIDOS prospective study. Lancet 1996; 348:511–4.

Harris ST, et al, Effects of estrone (ogen) on spinal bone density of postmenopausal women. Archives of Internal Medicine 1991; 151:1980–84.

Health and Public Policy Committee, American College of Physicians, Radiologic methods to evaluate bone mineral content. Annals of Internal Medicine 1984;100:908–11.

Henrich JB, Postmenopausal estrogen/breast cancer controversy. JAMA 1992;268:1985–90.

Hui SL, Slemenda CW, Johnston CC, Baseline measurement of bone mass predicts fracture in white women. Annals of Internal Medicine 1989; 111:335–361.

Jackson JA, Kleerekoper M, Osteoporosis in men: diagnosis, pathophysiology, and prevention. Medicine 1990;69:137–152.

Johnston CC, Slemenda CW, Melton LJ, Clinical use of bone densitometry. New England Journal of Medicine 1991;324:1105–9.

Karpf DB, et al, Prevention of nonvertebral fractures by alendronate. JAMA 1997;277:1159–64.

Kelepouris N, et al, Severe osteoporosis in men. Annals of Internal Medicine 1995;123:452.

174 — References

Klevay L, Evidence of dietary copper and zinc deficiencies. JAMA 1979; 241:1917–18.

Knapen MHJ, Effect of vitamin K supplementation on circulating osteocalcin and urinary calcium excretion. Annals of Internal Medicine 1989; 111:1001–05.

Lane NE, et al, Running, osteoarthritis, and bone density: initial 2-year longitudinal study. American journal of Medicine 1990;88:452–9.

Lee JR, Is natural progesterone the missing link in osteoporosis prevention and treatment? Medical Hypotheses 1991, Aug; 316–8.

Lee JR, Osteoporosis reversal with transdermal progesterone. Lancet 1990, Nov; 24:1327.

Lee, J, Natural Progesterone: Multiple roles of a remarkable hormone, BLL, Sebastopol, CA 1993.

Levine J, and Nelson D, Esophageal stricture associated with alendronate therapy. American Journal of Medicine 1997;102:489–91.

Liberman UA, et al, Effect of oral alendronate on bone mineral density and the incidence of fractures in postmenopausal osteoporosis. New England Journal of Medicine 1995;333:1437.

Lippuner K, et al, Prevention of postmenopausal bone loss using tibolone or conventional peroral or transdermal hormone replacement therapy with 17B-estradiol and dydrogesterone. Journal of Bone Mineral Research 1997;12:806–12.

Lufkin EG, et al, Treatment of postmenopausal osteoporosis with transdermal estrogen. Annals of Internal Medicine 1992;117:117–9.

Lufkin EG, et al, Raloxifene treatment of postmenopausal osteoporosis. Journal of Bone Mineral Research 1997; 12(suppl 1):S150.

Macintyre I, et al, Calcitonin for prevention of postmenopausal bone loss. Lancet 1988;1:900–1.

McPherson K, Breast cancer and hormonal supplements in postmenopausal women. BMJ 1995, Sept 16.

Melton LJ, et al, Long-term fracture prediction by bone mineral assessed at different skeletal sites. Journal of Bone Mineral Research 1993; 8:1227–33.

Melton LJ, et al, Perspective: how many women have osteoporosis? Journal of Bone Mineral Research 1992;7:1005–10.

Miller D, et al, Breast cancer before age 45 and oral contraceptive use: new findings. American Journal of Epidemiology 1989;129.2:269–80.

National Academy of Science. Recommended daily allowances (Washington, D.C.: National Academy of Sciences, 1989).

Nelson M, et al, Effects of high-intensity strength training on multiple risk factors for osteoporotic fractures: a randomized controlled trial. JAMA 1994;272.24:1909–14.

NIH Consensus Development Panel, Optimal calcium intake. JAMA 1994; 272.24:1942–8.

Nilsson BE, Westlin NE, Bone density in athletes. Clinical Orthopaedic and Related Research 1971;77:179–182.

Overgaard K, et al, Effect of salcatonin given intranasally on bone mass and fracture rates in established osteoporosis: a dose-response study. BMJ 1992;305:556–61.

Pak CYC, et al, Safe and effective treatment of osteoporosis with intermittent slow release sodium fluoride: augmentation of vertebral bone mass and inhibition of fractures. Journal of Clinical Endocrinology and Metabolism 1989, 68:150–9.

Pak CYC, et al, Treatment of postmenopausal osteoporosis with slow-release fluoride: final update of a randomized controlled trial. Annals of Internal Medicine 1995;123:401–8.

Pappoulos SE, et al, Use of bisphosphonates in the treatment of osteoporosis. Bone 1992; 13:

Parfitt A, Metabolic bone disease after intestinal bypass for treatment of obesity. Annals of Internal Medicine 1978;89:193–9.

Passeri M, et al, Effect of ipriflavone on bone mass in elderly osteoporotic women. Bone and Mineral 1992;19:S57–S62.

Petitti D, et al, Increased risk of cholecystectomy in users of supplemental estrogen. Gastroenterology 1988; 94:91–5.

Pollitzer WS, Anderson JJB, Ethnic and genetic differences in bone mass: a review with hereditary vs environmental perspective. American Journal Clinical Nutrition 1989;50:1244–59.

Powles TJ, et al, Effect of tamoxifen on bone mineral density measured by dual-energy X-ray absorptiometry in healthy premenopausal and postmenopausal women. Journal of Clinical Oncology 1996;14:78–84.

Price EH, et al, Women need to be warned about dangers of hormone replacement therapy. British Medical Journal 1997;314:376–7.

Prior J, et al, Progesterone and the Prevention of osteoporosis, Can J OB/ GYN 1991;3(4):181–6.

Randall T, Longitudinal study pursues questions of calcium, hormones, and metabolism in life of skeleton. JAMA 1992;268.17:2353–7.

Reginster JY, Management of high turnover osteoporosis with calcitonin. Bone 1992;S41–9.

Reginster JY, et al, One-year controlled randomized trial of prevention of early postmenopausal bone loss by intranasal calcitonin. Lancet 1987;2:1481–3.

Riggs BL, Melton LJ, 3d. Prevention and treatment of osteoporosis. New England Journal of Medicine 1992;327:620.

Riggs BL, et al, Effect of fluoride treatment on fracture rate in postmeno- pausal women with osteoporosis. New England Journal of Medicine 1990;322:802–9.

Rubin SM, Cummings SR, Results of bone densitometry affect women's decisions about taking measures to prevent fractures. Annals of Internal Medicine 1992;116:990–5.

Rymer J, et al, Effect of tibolone on postmenopausal bone loss. Osteoporo- sis International 1994;4:314–9.

Shangold MM, Exercise in the menopausal woman. Obstetrics and Gyne- cology 1990;75:53S–8S.

Sinaki M, Mikkelson BA, Postmenopausal spinal osteoporosis: flexion versus extension exercises. Archives of Physical Medicine and Rehabilita- tion 1984;65:593–6.

Slemenda CW, Christian JC, Reed T, Long-term bone loss in men: effects of genetic and environmental factors. Annals of internal Medicine 1992;117:286–91.

Slemenda C, et al, Predictors of bone mass in perimenopausal women. Annals of Internal Medicine 1990;112.2:96–101.

Slovik DM, et al, Deficient production of 1,25 dihydroxyvitamin D in elderly osteoporotic patients. New England Journal of Medicine 1981;305:372–4.

Soma MR, et al, Lowering of Lp[a] induced by estrogen plus progesterone replacement therapy in postmenopausal women, Arch Intern Med 1993 Jun 28;153(12):1462–8.

Stampfer M, et al, Postmenopausal estrogen therapy and cardiovascular disease: ten-year follow-up from the nurses study. New England Journal of Medicine 1991;325.11:756–761.

Stevenson JC, Pathogenesis, prevention, and treatment of osteoporosis. Obstetical Gynecology 1990;75.528:368–418.

Storm T, et al, Effect of intermittent cyclical etidronate therapy of bone mass and fracture rate in women with postmenopausal osteoporosis. New England Journal of Medicine 1990;322:1265–71.

Wasnich RD, et al, Prediction of Posmenopausal Fracture Risk with Use of Bone Mineral Measurements. American Journal of Obstetrics and Gynecology 1985;153:745–51.

Watts NB, et al, Intermittent Cyclical Etidronate Treatment of Postmenopausal Osteoporosis. New England Journal of Medicine. 1990;323:73–9.

Whitehead MI, et al, Effects of Estrogens and Progestins on the Biochemistry and Morphology of the Postmenopausal Endometrium. New England Journal of Medicine 1981;305:1599–1605.

Wingo PA, et al, The Risk of Breast Cancer in Postmenopausal Women Who Have Used Estrogen Replacement Therapy. JAMA 1987;257:209–15.

Yang S, et al, Radiographic Absorptiometry for Bone Mineral Measurement of the Phalanges: Precision and Accuracy Study. Radiology 1994;192:857–9.

Chapter 6

Anderson RL, Wolf WJ, Compositional changes in trypsin inhibitors, phytic acid, saponins, and isoflavones related to soybean processing. J Nutr 1995;125(3):581–6.

Funaba M, Hashimoto M, Yamanaka C, Shimogori Y, Iriki T, Ohshima S, Abe M, Effects of a high-protein diet on mineral and struvite activity product in clinically normal cats. Am J Vet Res 1996;57(12):1726–32.

Feskanich D, Willett WC, Stampfer MJ, Colditz GA, Protein consumption and bone fractures in women. Am J Epidemiol 1996;143(5):472–9.

Cooper C, Atkinson EJ, Hensrud DD, Wahner HW, O'Fallen WM, Riggs BL, Melton LD 3rd, Dietary protein intake and bone mass in women. Calcif Tissue Int 1996;58(5):320–5.

Eaton-Evans J, Osteoporosis and the role of diet. Br J Biomed Sci 1994;51(4):358–70.

Hosokawa M, Yanagi H, Kawanami K, Tanaka K, Kobayashi K, Amagai H,

Tmura S, Tsuchiya S, Relationship between dietary lifestyle in youth and osteoporosis. Nippon Koshu Eisei Zasshi 1996;43(8):606–14.

Marsh AG, Sanchez TV, Michelsen O, Chaffee FL, Fagal SM, Vegetarian lifestyle and bone mineral density. Am J Clin Nutr 1988;48 (3 Suppl):837–41.

Adlercreutz H, Mazur W, Phytoestrogens and Western diseases, Ann Med 1997;29(2):95–120.

Omi N, Aooi S, Murata K, Ezawa I, Evaluation of the effect of soybean milk peptide on bone metabolism in the rat model with ovariectomized osteoporosis. J Nutr Sci Vitaminol 1994;40(2):201–11.

Knight DC, Eden JA, Phytoestrogens: a short review. Maturitas 1995;22(3):167–75.

Arjmandi BH, Alekel L, Hollis BW, Amin D, Staciwicz-Sapuntzakis M, Guo P, Kukreja SC, Dietary soybean protein prevents bone loss in an ovariectomized rat model of osteoporosis. J Nutr 1996;126(1):161–7.

Knight DC, Eden JA, A review of the clinical effects of phytoestrogens. Obstet Gynecol 1996;87(5 Pt 2):897–904.

Kurzer MS, Xu X, Dietary phytoestrogens. Annu Rev Nutr 1997;17:353–81.

Lien LL, Lien EJ, Hormone therapy and phytoestrogens. J Clin Pharm Ther 1996;21(2):101–11.

Sathos TH, Shulman RJ, Schanler RJ, Abrams SA, Effect of carbohydrates on calcium adsorption in premature infants. Pediatr Res 1996;39 (4 Pt 1):666–70.

Trinidad TP, Wolever TM, Thompson LU, Availabiltiy of calcium for absorption in the small intestines and colon from diets containing available and unavailable carbohydrates: an in-vitro assessment. Int J Food Sci Nutr 1996;47(1):83–8.

Chonan O, Matsumoto K, Watanuki M, Effect of galactooligo saccharides on calcium absorption and preventing bone loss in ovariectomized rats. Biosci Biotechnol Biochem 1995;59(2):236–9.

Trichopoulo A, Georgiou E, Bassikos Y, Lipworth L, Lagiou P, Proukakis C, Trichopoulos D, Energy intake and monounsaturated fat in relation to bone mineral density among women and men in Greece. Prev Med 1997;26(3):395–400.

Hara H, Nagata M, Ohta A, Kasai T, Increases in calcium absorption with ingestion of soluble dietary fibre, guar-gum, hydrolysate, depends on the caecum in partially nephrectomized normal rats. Br J Nutr 1996;76(5):773–84.

Coudray C, Bellanger J, Castiglia-Delavaud C, Remesy C, Vermorel M, Rayssignuier Y, Effect of soluble or partly soluble fiber supplementation on absorption and balance of calcium, magnesium, iron, and zinc in healthy young men. Eur J Clin Nutr 1997;51(6):375–80.

Avenell A, Richmond PR, Lean ME, Reid DM, Bone loss associated with a high-fibre weight reduction diet in postmenopausal women. Eur J Clin Nutr 48(8):561–6.

Sasson A, Etzion Z, Shany S, Berlyne GM, Yagil R, Growth and bone mineralisation as affected by dietary calcium, phytic acid and vitamin D. Comp Biochem Physiol 1982;72(1):43–8.

Chanda S, Islam MN, Pramanik P, Mitra C, High-lipid intake is a possible predisposing factor in the development of hypogonadal osteoporosis. Jpn J Physiol 1996;46(5):383–8.

Parhami F, Morrow AD, Balucan J, Leitinger N, Watson AD, Tintut Y, Berliner JA, Demer LL, Lipid oxidation products have opposite effects on calcifying vascular cell and bone cell differentiation: a possible explanation for the paradox of arterial calcification in osteoporotic patients. Arterioscler Thromb Vasc Biol 1997;17(4):680–7.

Owen RW, Weisgerber UM, Carr J, Harrison MH, Analysis of calcium-lipid complexes in feces. Eur J Cancer Prev 1995;4(3):247–55.

Goulding A, McIntosh J, Effects of NaCl on calcium balance, parathyroid function and hydroxyproline excretion in prednisolone-treated rats consuming low-calcium diet. J Nutr 1986;116(6):37–44.

Greendale GA, Barrett-Connor E, Edelstein S, Ingles S, Haile R, Dietary sodium and bone mineral density; result of a 16-year follow-up study. J Am Geriatr Soc 1994;42(10):1050–5.

Dawson-Hughes B, Fowler SE, Dalsky G, Gallagher C, Sodium excretion influences calcium homeostasis in elderly men and women. J Nutr 1996;126(9):2107–12.

Antonios TF, MacGregor GA, Deleterious effects of salt intake other than effects on blood pressure. Clin Exp Pharmacol Physiol 1995;22(3):180–4.

Barger-Lux MJ, Heaney RP, Caffeine and the calcium economy revisited. Osteoporosis Int 1995;5(2):97-102.

Wise KJ, Bergman EA, Sherrard DJ, Massey LK, Interactions between dietary calcium and caffeine consumption on calcium metabolism in hypertensive humans. Am J Hypertens 1996;9(3):223–9.

Harris SS, Dawson-Hughes B, Caffeine and bone loss in healthy postmenopausal women. Am J Clin Nutr 1994;60(4):573–8.

Packard PT, Recker RR, Caffeine does not affect the rate of gain in spine bone in young women. Osteoporosis Int 1994;6(2):149–52.

Lloyd T. Rollins N, Eggli DF, Kieselhorst K, Chinchilli VM, Dietary caffeine intake and bone status of postmenopausal women. Am J Clin Nutr 1997;65(6):1826–30.

Faine MP, Dietary factors related to preservation of oral and skeletal bone mass in women. J Prosthet Dent 1995;73(1):65–72.

Ferrini RL, Barrett-Connor E, Caffeine intake and sex steroid levels in postmenopausal women. The Rancho Bernardo Study. Am J Epidemiol 1996;144(7):642–4.

Hintz HF, Calcium, cola, calamity. Cornell Vet 1980;70(1):3–9.

Calvo MS, The effects of high phosphorus intake on calcium homeostasis. Adv Nutr Res 1994;9:183–207.

Wyshak G, Frisch RE, Carbonated beverages, dietary calcium, the calcium/phosphorus ratio, and bone fractures in girls and boys. J Adolesc Health 1994;15(3):210–5.

Kimble RB, Alcohol, cytokines, and estrogens in the control of bone remodeling. Alcohol Clin Exp Res 1997;21(3):385–91.

Keller ET, Zhang J, Ershler WB, Ethanol activates the interleukin-6 promoter in a human marrow stromal cell line. J Gerontol A Biol Sci 1997;52(6):B311–7.

Laitinen K, Tiahtalla R, LuomanmIaki K, VialimIaki MJ, Mechanisms of hypocalcemia and markers of bone turnover in alcohol-intoxicated drinkers. Bone Miner 1994;24(3):171–9.

McCaughan GW, Feller RB, Osteoporosis in chronic liver disease: pathogenesis, risk factors, and management. Dig Dis 1994;12(4):223–31.

Felson DT, Zhang Y, Hannan MT, Kannel WB, Kiel DP, Alcohol intake and bone mineral density in elderly men and women. The Framingham Study. Am J Epidemiol 1995;142(5):485–92.

Abbott L, Nadler J, Rude RK, Magnesium deficiency in alcoholism: possible contribution to osteoporosis and cardiovascular disease in alcoholics. Alcohol Clin Exp Res 1994;18(5):1076–82.

Sarli M, Plotkin H, Zanchetta JR, Alcoholic osteopathy. Medicina (B aries) 1994;54(4):63–70.

Haugeberg G, Osteoporosis in rheumatoid arthritis. Tidsskr Nor Laegeforen 1997;117(5):651–4.

Ringe JD. Generalized osteoporosis in chronic polyarthritis-pathomechanisms and treatment approaches, A Rheumatol 1996;55(3):149–57.

Skerry TM, The effects of the inflammatory response on bone growth. Eur J Clin Nutr 1994;48 Suppl 1: S190–7.

Breil L, Koch T, Heller A, Schlotzer E, Grunert A, van Ackern K, Neuhof H, Alteration of n-3 fatty acid composition in lung tissue after short-term infusion of fish oil emulsion attenuates inflammatory vascular reaction. Crit Care Med 1996;24(11):1893–902.

Blok WL, Katan MB, van der Meer JW, Modulation of inflammation and cytokine production by dietary n-3 fatty acids. J Nutr 1996;126(6):1515–33.

Manolagas SC, Jika RL, Bone marrow, cytokines, and bone remodeling: emerging insights into the pathophysiology of osteoporosis. N Eng J Med 1995;332(5):305–11.

Linz DN, Garcia VF, Arya G, Ziegler MM, Prostaglandin and tumor necrosis factor levels in early wound inflammatory fluid: effects of parenteral omega-3 and omega-6 fatty acid administration. J Pediatr Surg 1994;29(8):1065–9.

De Caterina R, Cybulsky MI, Clinton SK, Gimbrone MA, Libby P, The omega-3 fatty acid docosahexanoate reduces cytokine-induced expression of proatherogenic and proinflammatory proteins in human endothelial cells. Arterioscler Thromb 1994;14(11):1829–36.

Sakaguchi K, Morita I, Murota S, Eicosapentaenoic acid inhibits loss due to ovariectomy rats. Prostaglandins Leukot Essent Fatty Acids, 50(2):81–4.

Krener JM. Effects of modulation of inflammatory and immune parameters in patients with rheumatic and inflammatory disease receiving dietary supplementation of n-3 and n-6 fatty acids. Lipids 1996;31 Suppl: S243–7.

Wachtler P, Konig W, Senkal M, Koller M, Influence of a total parenteral nutrition enriched with omega-3 fatty acids on leukotriene synthesis of peripheral leukocytes and systemic cytokine levels in patients with major surgery. J Trauma 1997;42(2):191–8.

Das UN, Beneficial effect of eicosapentaenoic and docosahexanoic acids in the management of sytemic lupus erythematosus and its relationship to the cytokine network. Prostaglandins Leukot Essent Fatty Acids 1994;51(3): 207–13.

Struijs A, Mulder H, The effects of inhaled glucocorticoids on bone mass and biochemical markers of bone homeostasis: a 1-year study of beclothasone versus budesonide. Neth J Med 1997;50(6):233–7.

Peacey SR, Guo CY, Robinson AM, Price A, Giles MA, Eastell R, Weetman AP, Glucocorticoid replacement therapy: are patients overtreated and does it matter? Clin Endocrinol 1997;46(3):255–61.

Reid IR, Veale AG, France JT, Glucocorticoid osteoporosis. J Asthma 1994;31(1):7–18.

Delaney AM, Dong Y, Canalis E, Mechanisms of glucocorticoid action in bone cells. J Cell Biochem 56(3):295–302.

Adler RA, Rosen CJ, Glucocorticoids and osteoporosis. Endocrinol Metab Clin North Am 1994;23(3):641–51.

Sarne DH, Thyroid hormone effects on bone and thyroid disorders. Crisp Data Base National Institute of Health, 1996.

L'imanov'a Step'an J, The risk for osteoporosis in persons treated with thyroid hormones. Vnitr Lek 1992;38(9):860–7.

Schneider DL, Barrett O, Connor EL, Morton DL, Thyroid hormone use and bone mineral density in elderly men. Arch Intern Med 1995;155(18):2005–7.

Nuovo J, Ellsworth A, Christensen DB, Reynolds R, Excessive thyroid hormone replacement therapy. J Am Board Fam Pract 1995;8(6):435–9.

Franklyn JA, Betteridge J, Holder R, Oates GD, Parle JV, Lilley J, Heath DA, Sheppard MC, Long-term thyroxine treatment and bone mineral density. Lancet 1992;340(8810):9–13.

Bisbocci D, Gallo V, Damiano P, Sidoli L, Cantoni R, Aimo G, Priolo G, Pagni R, Chiandussi L, Spontaneous release of interleukin-1 beta from human blood monocytes in thyrotoxic osteodystrophy. J Endocrinol Invest, 1996;19(8):511–5.

Schneider DL, Barrett-Connor EL, Morton DL, Thyroid hormone use and bone mineral density in elderly women: effect of estrogen. JAMA 1994;271(16):1245–9.

Murray WJ, Lindo VS, Kakkar VV, Melissari E, Long-term administration of heparin and heparin fractions and osteoporosis in experimental animals. Blood Coagul Fibrinolysis 1995;6(2):113–8.

Chigot P, De Gennes C, Samama MM, Osteoporosis induced either by unfractionated heparin or by low-molecular-weight heparin. J Mal Vasc 1996;21(3):121–5.

Sivakumaran M, Ghosh K, Zaidi Y, Hutchinson RM, Osteoporosis and vertebral collapse following low-dose, low-molecular weight. Clin Lab Haematol 1996;18(1):55–7.

Barbour LA, Kick SD, Steiner JF, LoVerde ME, Heddleston LN, Lear JL, Barion AE, Barton PL, A prospective study of heparin-induced osteoporosis in pregnancy using bone densitometry. Am J Obstet Gynecol 1994;170(3):862–9.

Panagakos FS, Jandinski JJ, Feder L, Kumar S, Heparin fails to potentiate the effects of IL-1 beta-mediated bone resorption of fetal rat bones in vitro. Biochimie 1995;77(12):915–8.

Bergqvist D, Low-molecular-weight heparins. J Intern Med 1996; 240(2):63–72.

Ensminger AH, Ensminger ME, Konlande JE, Robson JRK, The Concise Encyclopedia of Foods & Nutrition. Boca Raton, FL: CRC Press;1995.

Mahan KL, Escott-Stump S, Food, Nutrition and Diet Therapy 9th edition, Philadelphia, PA: WB Saunders; 1996.

Brandi, ML, Natural and synthetic isoflavones in the prevention and treatment of chronic diseases. Calcif Tissue Int 1997;61 Suppl 1:S5–8.

Anderson, JB, et al, The effects of phytoestrogens on bone. Nutrition Research 1997;17(10):1617–32.

Knight, DC, et al, A review of the clinical effects of phytoestrogens. Obstet Gynecol 1996, May;87(5 Pt 2):897–904.

Barnes, S, Evolution of the health benefits of soy isoflavones. Proc Soc Exp Biol Med 1998, Mar;217(3):386–92.

Clarkson, TB, et al, Estrogenic soybean isoflavones and chronic disease: risks and benefits. Trends Endocrinol Metab 1995;6:11–16.

Hughes, CL, Phytochemical mimicry of reproductive hormones and modulation of herbivore fertility of phytoestrogens. Environ Health Perspect 1988;78:171–5.

Wilcox, G, et al, Oestrogenic effects of plant foods in postmenopausal women. BMJ 1990;30:905–6.

Potter, SM, et al, Soy protein and isoflavones: their effects on blood lipids and bone density in postmenopausal women. AM J Clin Nutr 1998 (in press).

Anderson, JB, et al, Biphasic effects of genistein on bone tissue in the ovariectomized, lactating rat model. Proc Soc Biol Med 1997.

Cassidy, A, et al, Biological effects of a diet of soy protein rich in isoflavones on the menstrual cycle of postmenopausal women. Am J Clin Nutr 1994;60:333–40.

Blair, HC, et al, Variable effects of tyrosine kinase inhibitors on ovarian osteoclastic activity and reduction of bone loss in ovariectomized rats. J Cell Biochem 1996;61:620–37.

Ishida, H, et al, Preventive effects of the plant isoflavones, daidzein and genistein, on bone loss in ovariectomized rats fed a calcium-deficient diet. Biol Pharm Bull 1998, Jan;21(1):62–6.

Verdeal, K, et al, Naturally occurring estrogen plant foodstuffs: a review. J Food Prot 1979;42:577–83.

Cassidy, A, et al, Biological effects of plant estrogens in postmenopausal women. Fed AM Soc Exp Biol 1993;7(abst):A866.

Anderson, JB, et al, The effects of phytoestrogens on bone, Nutrition Research 1997;17 (10) 1617–32.

Knight, DC, et al, A review of the clinical effects of phytoestrogens, Obstet Gynecol 1996, May;87(5 Pt 2):897–904.

Barnes, S, Evolution of the health benefits of soy isoflavones, Proc Soc Exp Biol Med 1998, Mar;217(3):386–92.

Anderson, JB, et al, Phytoestrogens and human function. Nutrition Today 1997; 32(6): 232–9.

Clarkson, TB, et al, Estrogenic soybean isoflavones and chronic disease: risks and benefits. Trends Endocrinol Metab 1995;6:11–16.

Wilcox, G, et al, Oestrogenic effects of plant foods in postmenopausal women. BMJ 1990;30:905–6.

Adlercreutz, H, et al, Dietary phytoestrogen and menopause in Japan. Lancet,

Draper CR, et al, Phytoestrogens reduce bone loss and bone resorption in oophorectomized rats. J Nutr, 1997;127 (9):1795–9.

Anderson JJ, Ambrose WW, Garner SC, Biphasic effects of genistein on bone tissue in the ovariectomized lactating rat model. Proc Soc Exp Biol Med 1998;217(3):345–50.

Arjmandi BH, Alekel L, et al, Dietary soybean protein prevents bone loss in an ovariectomized rat model of osteoporosis. J Nutr 1996;126(1):161–7.

Chapter 7

Nordin BE, Calcium and osteoporosis. Nutrition 1997, Jul–Aug;13(7-8):664–86.

Quantock C, et al, The role of calcium and vitamin D in osteoporosis. Community Nurse 1996, Sep;2(8):48–9.

Cayon E, et al, Solubility of calcium salts and their effects on osteoporosis. Methods Find Exp Clin Pharmacol 1997, Sep;19(7):501–4.

Fukuda S, et al, Intestinal calcium absorption and response of calcium regulating hormones in the stroke-prone spontaneously hypertensive rat as a model of osteoporosis. Clin Exp Pharmacol Physiol Suppl 1995;1:S240–1.

Reid IR, Therapy of osteoporosis: calcium, vitamin D and exercise. Am J Med Sci 1996, Dec;312(6):278–86.

Tellez M, et al, Gastrointestinal calcium absorption and dietary calcium load: relationships with bone remodelling in vertebral osteoporosis. Osteoporosis Int 1995, Jan;5(1):14–22.

Scopacasa F., et al, Calcium supplementation suppresses bone resorption in early postmenopausal women. Calcif Tissue Int 1998, Jan;62(1):8–12.

Need AG, et al, Biochemical effects of a calcium supplement in osteoporotic postmenopausal women with normal absorption and malabsorption of calcium. Miner Electrolyte Metab 1987;13(2):112–6.

Dawson-Hughes, B, et al, Effect of calcium and vitamin D supplementation on bone density in men and women 65 years of age or older. N Engl J Med 1997, Sep 4;337(10):670–6.

Recker R, Calcium absorption and achlorhydria, NEJM 1985;313:70–3.

Erlacher L, et al, Salmon calcitonin and calcium in the treatment of male osteoporosis: the effect on bone mineral density. Wien Klin Wochenschr 1997, Apr 25;109(8):270–4.

Schauss A, Colloidal minerals: clinical implications of clay suspension products sold as dietary supplements. Am J Natural Med 1977;4(1):5–10.

Reid IR, et al, Therapy of osteoporosis: calcium, vitamin D and exercise. Am J Med Sci 1996, Dec;312(6):278–86.

Bourgoin BP, et al, Lead content of 70 brands of dietary calcium supplements. Am J Public Health 1993;83:1155–60.

Kaufman JM, et al, Role of calcium and vitamin D in the prevention and treatment of postmenopausal osteoporosis: an overview. Clin Rheumatol 1995, Sep;14 Suppl 3:9–13.

Halpern GM, et al, Comparative uptake of calcium from milk and a calcium-rich mineral water in lactose intolerant adults: implications for the treatment of osteoporosis. Am J Prev Med 1991, Nov-Dec;7(6):379–83.

Wynckel A et al, Intestinal calcium absorption from mineral water. Miner Electrolyte Metab 1977;23(2):88–92.

Sardana R, et al, Nutritional management of osteoporosis. Geriatr Nurs 1992, Nov–Dec;13(6):315–9.

Shiraki M, Calcium metabolism and osteoporosis. Nippon Naika Gakkai Zasshi 1992, Sep 10;81(9):1392–6.

Heaney RP, Calcium in the prevention and treatment of osteoporosis. J Intern Med 1992, Feb;231(2):169–80.

Wallach S, Relation of magnesium to osteoporosis and calcium urolithiasis. Magnes Trace Elem 1991–2;10(2-4):281–6.

Whiting SJ, Calcium supplementation. J Am Acad Nurse Pract 1977, Apr;9(4):187–92.

Devine A, et al, A 4-year follow-up study of the effects of calcium supplementation on bone density in elderly postmenopausal women. Osteoporosis Int 1997;7(1):23–8.

Blumsohn A, et al, The effect of calcium supplementation on the circadian rhythm of bone resorption. J Clin Endocrinol Metab 1994, Sep;79(3):730–5.

Leveille SG, et al, Dietary vitamin C and bone mineral density in postmenopausal women in Washington state, J Epidemiol Community Health 1997 Oct;51(5):479–85.

Murray TM, Prevention and management of osteoporosis: consensus statements from the Scientific Advisory Board of the Osteoporosis Society of Canada. CMAJ 1996, Oct 1;155(7):935–9.

Arnaud CD, et al, The role of calcium in osteoporosis. Annu Rev Nutr 1990;10:397–414.

Coudray C, et al, Effect of soluble or partly soluble dietary fiber supplementation on absorption and balance of calcium, magnesium, iron and zinc in healthy young men. Eur J Clin Nutr 1997, Jun;(51)(6):375–80.

Sojka JE, et al, Magnesium supplementation and osteoporosis. Nutr Rev 1995, Mar;53(3):71–4.

Rude RK, et al, Magnesium deficiency: possible role in osteoporosis with gluten sensitive enteropathy. Osteoporosis Int 1996;6(6):453–61.

Abbott L, et al, Magnesium deficiency in alcoholism: possible contribution to osteoporosis and cardiovascular disease in alcoholics. Alcohol Clin Exp Res 1994, Oct;18(5):1076–82.

Stendig-Lindberg G, et al, Trabecular bone density in a two-year controlled trial of peroral magnesium in osteoporosis. Magnes Res 1993, Jun;6(2):155–63.

Steidl L, et al, Osteoporosis treated with magnesium lactate. Acta Univ Palacki Olomuc Fac Med 1991;129:99–106.

Wallach S, Relation of magnesium to osteoporosis and calcium urolithiasis. Magnes Trace Elem 1991;10(2-4):281–6.

Steidl L, et al, Blood magnesium, calcium and zinc in osteoporosis. Acta Univ Palacki Olomuc Fac Med 1991;129:91–8.

Seelig MS, Increased need for magnesium with the use of combined estrogen and calcium for osteoporosis treatment. Magnes Res 1990, Sep;3(3):197–215.

Steidl L, et al, Blood magnesium findings in osteoporosis. Acta Univ Palacki Olomuc Fac Med 1990;126:117–28.

Matsuda Y, et al, Effect of magnesium sulfate treatment on neonatal bone abnormalities. Gynecol Obstet Invest 1997;44(2):82–8.

Vormann J, et al, Effects of magnesium deficiency on magnesium and calcium content in bone and cartilage in developing rats in correlation to chondrotoxicity. Calcif Tissue Int 1997, Sep;61(3):230–8.

Navarro JF, et al, Serum magnesium concentration and PTH levels. Scand J Urol Nephrol 1997, Jun;31(3):275–80.

Heubi, JE et al, The role of magnesium in the pathogenesis of bone disease in childhood cholestatic liver disease. J Pediatr Gastroenterol Nutr 1997, Sep;(25(3):301–6.

Schanler RJ, et al, Effects of long-term maternal intravenous magnesium sulfate therapy on neonatal calcium metabolism and bone mineral content. Gynecol Obstet Invest 1997;43(4):236–41.

Cohen L, et al, Infrared spectroscopy and magnesium content of bone mineral in osteoporotic women. Isr J Med Sci 1981;17:1123–5.

Jones G, et al, Prevention and management of osteoporosis: vitamin D metabolites and analogs in the treatment of osteoporosis. CMAJ 1996, Oct 1;155(7):955–61.

Tamai M, et al, Correlation between vitamin D receptor genotypes and bone mineral density in Japanese patients with osteoporosis. Calcif Tissue Int 1997, Mar;60(3):229–32.

Ringe JD, Active vitamin D metabolites in glucocorticoid-induced osteoporosis. Calcif Tissue Int 1997, Jan;60(1):124–7.

Bonjour JP, et al, Nutritional aspects of hip fractures. Bone 1996 Mar;18 Suppl 3:139S–144S.

Schlagheck TG, et al, Olestra's effect on vitamins D and E in humans can be offset by increasing dietary levels of these vitamins. J Nutr 1997, Aug;127(Suppl 8):1666S–85S.

Heaney RP, et al, Calcium absorptive effects of vitamin D and its major metabolites. J Clin Endocrinolo Metab 1997, Dec;82(12):4111–6.

Lips P, Vitamin D deficiency and osteoporosis: the role of vitamin D deficiency and treatment with vitamin D and analogs in the prevention of osteoporosis-related fractures. Eur J Clin Invest 1996, Jun;(26(6):436–42.

Gallagher JC, The role of vitamin D in the pathogenesis and treatment of osteoporosis. J Rheumatol Suppl 1996, Aug;45:15–8.

Adachi JD, Vitamin D and calcium in the prevention of corticosteroid-induced osteoporosis. J Rheumatol 1996, Jun;23(6):995–1000.

Kaufman JM, Role of calcium and vitamin D in the prevention and the treatment of postmenopausal osteoporosis: an overview. Clin Rheumatol 1995, Sep;14 Suppl 3:9–13.

Fujita T, Vitamin D in the treatment of osteoporosis revisited. Proc Soc Exp Biol Med 1996, Jun;212(2):110–5.

Peris P, et al, Etiology and presenting symptoms in male osteoporosis. Br J Rheumatol 1995, Oct;34(10):936–41.

Nordin BE, Osteoporosis and vitamin D. J Cell Biochem 1992, May;49(1): 19–25.

Dawson-Hughes B, et al, Rates of bone loss in postmenopausal women randomly assigned to one of two dosages of vitamin D. Am J Clin Nutr 1995;61:1140–45.

Ooms ME, et al, Prevention of bone loss by vitamin D supplementation in elderly women. J Clin Endocrinol Metabol 1995;80:1052–58.

Chapuy MC, et al, Effect of calcium and cholecalciferol treatment for three years on hip fractures in elderly women. BMJ 1994;308:1081–82.

Dambacher MA, et al, Can the fast bone loss in osteoporotic and osteopenic patients be stopped with active vitamin D metabolites? Calcif Tissue Int 1997, Jan;60(1):115–8.

Holick MF, Environmental factors that influence the cutaneous production of vitamin D. Am J Clin Nutr 1995, Mar;61Suppl 3:638S–645S.

Binkly NC, et al, Vitamin K nutrition and osteoporosis. J Nutr 1995, Jul;125(7):1812–21.

Kaneki M, et al, Serum concentrations of vitamin K in elderly women with involutional osteoporosis. Nippon Ronen Igakkai Zasshi 1995, Mar;32(3):195–200.

Weber P, Management of osteoporosis: is there a role for vitamin K? Int J Vitam Nutr Res 1997;67(5):350–6.

Douglas AS, Carboxylation of osteocalcin in postmenopausal women following vitamin K and D supplementation. Bone 1995, Jul;17(1):15–20.

Jie KG, et al, Vitamin K status and bone mass in women with and without aortic atherosclerosis. Calcif Tissue Int 1996, Nov;59(5):352–6.

Vermeer C, et al, Effects of vitamin K on bone mass and bone metabolism. J Nutr 1996, Apr;126Suppl4:1187S–91S.

Tamatani M, et al, Decreased circulating levels of vitamin K and 25-hydroxyvitamin D in osteopenic elderly men. Metabolism 1998, Feb;47(2):195–9.

Hodges SJ, et al, Depressed levels of circulating menaquinones in patients with osteoporotic fractures of the spine and femoral neck. Bone 1991;12(6):387–9.

Kohlmeier M, et al, Transport of vitamin K to bone in humans. J Nutr 1996, Apr;124Suppl 4:1192S–6S.

Vermeer C, et al, Role of vitamin K in bone metabolism. Annu Rev Nutr 1995;15:1–22.

Lafforgue P, et al, Bone mineral density in patients given vitamin K antagonists. Rev Rhem Engl Ed 1997, Apr;64(4):249–54.

Shearer MJ, et al, Chemistry, nutritional sources, tissue distribution and metabolism of vitamin K with special reference to bone health. J Nutr 1996, Apr;126 Suppl 4:1181S–6S.

Booth SL, Skeletal functions of vitamin K-dependent proteins: not just for clotting anymore. Nutr Rev 1997, Jul;55(7):282–4.

Koshihara Y, et al, Vitamin K enhances osteocalcin accumulation in the extracellular matrix of human osteoblasts in vitro. J Bone Miner Res 1997, Mar;12(3):431–8.

Gijsbers BL, et al, Effect of food composition on vitamin K absorption in human volunteers. Br J Nutr 1996, Aug;76(2):223–9.

Relea P, et al, Zinc biochemical markers of nutrition and type 1 osteoporosis. Age Ageing 1995, Jul;24(4):303–7.

Herzberg M, et al, The effect of estrogen replacement therapy on zinc in serum and urine. Obstet Gynecol 1996, Jun;87(6):1035–40.

Okano T, Effects of essential trace elements on bone turnover in relation to osteoporosis. Nippon Rinsho 1996, Jan;54(1):148–54.

McKenna AA, et al, Zinc balance in adolescent females consuming a low or high calcium diet. Am J Clin Nutr 1997, May;65(5):1460–4.

Wood RJ, et al, High dietary calcium intake reduces zinc absorption and balance in humans. Am J Clin Nutr 1997, Jun;65(6):1803–9.

Yee CD, et al, The relationship of nutritional copper to the development of postmenopausal osteoporosis in rats. Biol Trace Elem res 1995, Apr;48(1):1–11.

Strain JJ, A reassessment of diet and osteoporosis—possible role for copper. Med Hypotheses 1988, Dec;27(4):333–8.

Kotkowiak L, Behavior of selected bioelements in women with osteoporosis. Ann Acad Ned Stetin 1997;43:225–38.

Olivares M, et al, Copper as an essential nutrient. Am J Clin Nutr 1996, May;63(5):791S–6S.

Chapter 8

Reginster JY, et al, Design for an ipriflavone multicenter European fracture study. Calcif Tissue Int 1997;61 Suppl 1:S28–32.

Jilka RL, et al, Increased osteoclast development after estrogen loss: mediation by interleukin 6. Science 1992; 257:88–91.

Oursler MJ, Avian osteoclasts as estrogen target cells. Proc Natl Acad Sci USA 1991;88:6613–7.

Pensler J, et al, Osteoclasts isolated from membranous bone in children exhibited nuclear estrogen and progesterone receptors. J Bone Miner Res 1990;5:797–802.

Melis GB, et al, Lack of any estrogenic effect of ipriflavone in postmenopausal women. J Endocrinol Invest 1992;15:755–61.

Yamazaki I, et al, Effect of ipriflavone on osteoporosis induced by ovariectomy in rats. J Bone Miner Res 1986;3:205–10.

Petilli M, et al, Interactions between ipriflavone and the estrogen receptor. Calcif Tissue Int 1995;56:160–5.

Caltagirone S, et al, Interaction with type II estrogen binding sites and antiproliferative activity of tamoxifen and quercetin in human non-small-cell lung cancer. Am J Respir Cell Mol Biol 1997;17:51–9.

Markiewicz L, et al, In vitro bioassays of non-steroidal phytoestrogens. J Steroid Biochem Mol Biol 1993;45:399–405.

Notoya K, et al, Inhibitory effect of ipriflavone on osteoclast mediated bone resorption and new osteoclast formation in long-term cultures of mouse unfractionated bone cells. Calcif Tissue Intl 1993;53:206–9.

Benvenuti S, et al, Binding and bioeffects of ipriflavone on a human preosteoclastic cell line. Biochem Biophys Res Comm 1994;201:1084–9.

Agnusdei D, et al, Short-term treatment of Paget's disease of bone with ipriflavone. Bone Miner 1992;19 Suppl 1:S35–42.

Mazzuoli G, et al, Effects of ipriflavone on bone remodeling in primary hyperparathyroidism. Bone Miner 1992;19 Suppl 1:S35–42.

Cecchini MG, et al, Ipriflavone inhibits bone resorption in intact and ovariectomized rats. Calcif Tissue Int 1997; 61 Suppl 1:S9–11.

Miyauchi A, et al, Novel ipriflavone receptors coupled to calcium influx regulate osteclast differentiation and function. Endocrinology 1996;137: 3544–50.

Cheng S-L, et al, Stimulation of human osteblast differentiation and function by ipriflavone and its metabolites. Calcif Tissue Int 1994;55:356–62.

Kakai Y, et al, Effect of ipriflavone on the differentiation and proliferation of osteogenic cells. Calcif Tissue Int 1992; 51 Suppl 1:S11–15.

Agnusdei D, et al, A double-blind, placebo-controlled trial of ipriflavone for prevention of postmenopausal spinal bone loss. Calcif Tissue Int 1997;61:142–7.

Adami S, et al, Ipriflavone prevents radial bone loss in postmenopausal women with low bone mass over 2 years. Osteoporosis Int 1997;7:119–25.

Agnusdei D, et al, Metabolic and clinical effects of ipriflavone on established postmenopausal osteoporosis. Drugs Exp Clin Res 1989;15: 97–104.

Agnusdei D, et al, Effects of ipriflavone on bone mass and bone remodeling in patients with established postmenopausal osteoporosis. Curr Ther Res 1992;51:82–91.

Bankova VS, et al, High-performance liquid chromatographic analysis of flavonoids from bee propolis. J Chromatogr 1982;242:135–43.

Monostory K, et al, The effects of ipriflavone and its main metabolites on theophylline biotransformation. Eur J Drug Metab Pharmacokinet 1996;21:61–6.

Valente M, et al, Effects of 1-year treatment with ipriflavone on bone in postmenopausal women with low bone mass. Calcif Tissue Int 1994;54:377–80.

Gambacciani M, et al, Effects of combined low dose of the isoflavone derivative ipriflavone and estrogen replacement on bone mineral density and metabolism in postmenopausal women. Maturitas 1997;28:75–81.

Arjmandi BH, et al, The ovarian hormone deficiency-induced hypercholesterolemia is reversed by soy protein and the synthetic isoflavone, ipriflavone. Nutr Res 1997;17:885–94.

Ushiroyama T, et al, Efficacy of ipriflavone and vitamin D therapy for the cessation of vertebral bone loss. Int J of Gynecology & Obstetrics 1995;48:283–8.

Agnusdei D, Bufalino L, Efficacy of ipriflavone in established osteoporosis and long-term safety. Calcif Tissue International, 1977; Suppl 1(61): PS23–7.

Ferenec L et al, Pharmacokinetics of ipriflavone. Acta Pharm Hung 1995, Nov;65(6):219–22.

Ferenec L, et al, Metabolism of ipriflavone. Acta Pharm Hung 1995, Nov;65(6):215–8.

Shino A, et al, Suppressive effect of ipriflavone on bone depletion in the experimental diabetic rat: dose response of ipriflavone. Life Sci 1988;42(11):1123–30.

Ozawa H, et al, Histochemical and fine structural study of bone in ipriflavone-treated rats. Calcif Tissue Int 1992;51 Suppl 1:S21–6.

Civitelli R, et al, Ipriflavone improves bone density and biochemical properties of adult male rat bones. Calcif Tissue Int 1995, Mar;56(3):215–9.

Notoya K, et al, Increase in femoral bone mass by ipriflavone alone and in combination with 1 alpha-hydroxyvitamin D3 in growing rats with skeletal unloading. Calcif Tissue Int 1996, Feb;58(2):88–94.

Ghezzo C, et al, Ipriflavone does not alter bone apatite crystal structure in adult male rats. Calcif Tissue Int 1996, Dec;59(6):496–9.

Takenaka M, et al, Effect of ipriflavone on bone changes induced by calcium-restricted, vitamin D-deficient diet in rats. Endocrinol Jpn 1986, Feb;33(1):23–7.

Chinoin Pharmaceutical and Chemical Works, Hungary, PCT Patent 09703664.

Yoshio K, Toshio K, Tamotsu N, Yuko MT, Shigeru S, Effect of ipriflavone and estrogen on the differentiation and proliferation of osteogenic cells. Calcif Tissue Int 1992;51 Suppl 1: S11–15.

Melis GB, et al, Ipriflavone and low doses of estrogens in the prevention of bone mineral loss in climacterium. Bone and Mineral 1992;19 Suppl: S49–56.

Attila BK, Overview of clinical studies with ipriflavone. Acta Pharm Hung 1995, Nov;65(6):223–8.

Agnusdei D, et al, Prevention of early postmenopausal bone loss using low doses of conjugated estrogens and the non-hormonal, bone-active drug ipriflavone. Osteoporosis Int 1995;5(6):462–6.

Cecchettin M, et al, Metabolic and bone effects after administration of ipriflavone and salmon calcitonin in postmenopausal women. Biomed Pharmacother 1995;49(10):465–8.

Gennari C, et al, Effect of chronic treatment with ipriflavone in postmenopausal women with low bone mass. Calcif Tissue Int 1997;61 Suppl 1:S19–22.

Nakamura S, et al, Effect of ipriflavone on bone mineral density and calcium-related factors in elderly females. Calcif Tissue Int 1992;51 Suppl 1:S30–4.

Chapter 9

Reid IR, Therapy of osteoporosis: calcium, vitamin D, and exercise. Am J Med Sci 1996;312(6):278–86.

Taggart HM, Connor SE, The relation of exercise habits to health beliefs and knowledge about osteoporosis. J Am Coll Health 1995;44(3):127–130.

Preisinger E, Alacamlioglu Y, Pils K, Bosina E, Metka M, Schneider B, Ernst E, Exercise therapy for osteoporosis: results of a randomised controlled trial. Br J Sports Med 1996;30(3):209–12.

Greendale GA, Barrett-Connor E, Edelstein S, Ingles S, Haile R, Lifetime leisure exercise and osteoporosis. The Rancho Bernardo study. Am J Epidemiol 1995;141(10):951–9.

Nakatsuka K, Kawakami H, Miki T. Exercise and physical therapy in osteo-porosis. Nippon Rinsho 1994;52(9):2360–6.

Drinkwater BL, Exercise in the prevention of osteoporosis. Osteopros Int 1993;3(1):169–71.

Gutin B, Kasper MJ, Can vigorous exercise play a role in osteoporosis prevention? A review. Osteoporos Int 1992;2(2):55–69.

Dalsky GP, The role of exercise in the prevention of osteoporosis. Compr Ther 1989;15(9):30–7.

Birge SJ, Dalsky G, The role of exercise in preventing osteoporosis. Public Health Rep 1989;104:54–8.

Disen G, Berker C, Oral A, Varan G, The role of physical exercise in prevention and management of osteoporosis. Clin Rheumatol 1989;8(2):70–5.

Ebrahim S, Thompson PW, Baskaran V, Evans K, Randomized placebo-controlled trial of brisk walking in the prevention of postmenopausal osteoporosis. Age Ageing 1997;26(4):253–60.

Kohrt WM, Ehsani AA, Birge SJ Jr, Effects of exercise involving predomi-nantly either joint-reaction or ground-reaction forces on bone mineral density in older women. J Bone Miner Res 1997;12(8):1253–61.

Bravo G, Gauthier P, Roy PM, Payette H, Gaulin P, Harvey M, Peloquin L, Dubois MF, Impact of a 12-month exercise program on the physical and psychological health of osteoporotic women. J Am Geriatr Soc 1996;44(7):756–62.

Preisinger E, Alacamlioglu Y, Pils K, Saradeth T, Schneider B, Therapeutic exercise in the prevention of bone loss. A controlled trial with women after menopause. Am J Phys Med Rehabil 1995;74(2):120–3.

Lanyon LE, Using functional loading to influence bone mass and architec-ture: objectives, mechanism, and relationships with estrogen of the mechanically adaptive process in bone. Bone 1996;181(1):37S–43S.

Prior JC, Barr SI, Chow R, Faulkner RA, Prevention and management of osteoporosis: consensus statements from the Scientific Advisory Board of the Osteoporosis Society of Canada. 5. Physical activity as therapy for osteoporosis. CMAJ 1996;155(7):940–4.

Barlet JP, Coxam V, Davicco MJ, Physical exercise and the skeleton. Arch Physiol Biochem 1995;103(6):681–98.

Braith RW, Mills RM, Welsch MA, Keller JW, Pollock ML, Resistance exercise training restores bone mineral density in heart transplant recipients. J AM Coll Cardiol 1996;28(6):1471–7.

Swedish Council on Technology Assessment in Health Care, Bone density measurement: a systematic review. J Intern Med Suppl 1997;739():1–60.

Lord SR, Ward JA, Williams P, Zivanovic E, The effects of a community exercise program on fracture risk factors in older women. Osteoporosis Int 1996; 6(5):361–7.

Lohman T, Going S, Pameter R, Hall M, Boyden T, Houtlkooper L, Ritenbaugh C, Bare L, Hill A, Aickin M, Effects of resistance training on regional and total bone mineral density in premenopausal women: a randomized prospective study. J Bone Miner Res 1995;10(7):1015–24.

Korht WM, Snead DB, Slatopolsky E, Birge SJ Jr, Additive effects of weight-bearing exercise and estrogen on bone mineral density on older women. J Bone Miner Res 1995;10(9):1303–11.

Berard A, Bravo G, Gauthier P, Meta-analysis of the effectiveness of physical activity for the prevention of bone loss in postmenopausal women. Osteoporos Int 1997;7(4):331–7.

Heinonen A, Kannus P, Sievanen H, Oja P, Pasanen M, Rinne M, IisiRasi K, Vuori I, Randomized controlled trial of effect of high-impact exercise on selected risk factors for osteoporotis fractures. Lancet 1996;348(9038):1343–7.

Morris Fl, Naughton GA, Gibbs JL, Carlson JS, Wark JD, Prospective ten-month exercise intervention in premarchal girls: positive effects on bone and lean mass. J Bone Miner Res 1997;12(9):1453–62.

Hartard M, Haber P, Ilieva D, Preisinger E, Siedl G, Huber J, Systematic strength training as a model of therapeutic intervention. A controlled trial in postmenopausal women with osteopenia. Am J Phys Med Rehabil 1996;75(1):21–8.

Taunton JE, Martin AD, Rhodes EC, Wolski LA, Donelly M, Elliot J, Exercise for the older woman: choosing the right prescription. Br J Sports Med 1997;31(1):5–10.

Eikien PA, Physical activity and bone mineral content in postmenopausal women. Ugeskr Laeger 1995;157(37):5086–91.

Zerath E, Holy X, Douce P, Guezennec CY, Chatard JC, Effect of endurance training on postexercise parathyroid hormone levels in elderly men. Med Sci Sports Exerc 1997;29(9):1139–45.

Kudlacek S, Pietschmann F, Bernecker P, Resch H, Willvonseder R, The impact of a senior dancing program on spinal and peripheral bone mass. Am J Phys Med Rehabil 1997;76(6):477–81.

Brahm H, Piehl-Aulin K, Ljunghall S, Biochemical markers of bone metabolism during distance running in healthy, regular-exercising men and women. Scand J Med Sci Sports 1996;6(1):26–30.

Thorsen K, Kristofferson A, Lorentzon R, The effects of brisk walking on markers of bone and calcium metabolism in postmenopausal women. Calcif Tissue Int 1996;58(4):221–5.

Bennell KL, Malcolm SA, Khan KM, Thomas SA, Reid SJ, Brukner PD, Ebeling PR, Wark JD, Bone mass and bone turnover in power athletes, endurance athletes, and controls: a 12-month longitudinal study. Bone 1997;20(5):477–84.

Swezey RL, Exercise for osteoporosis: is walking enough? The case for site-specific and resistive exercise. Spine 1996;21(23):2809–13.

Price JS, Jackson B, Eastell R, Wilson AM, Russel RG, Lanyon LE, Goodship AE, The response of the skeleton to physical training: a biochemcial study in horses. Bone 1995;17(3):221–7.

Caballero MJ, Mahedero G, Hernandez R, Alvarez JL, Rodriquez J, Rodriguez I, Maynar M, Effects of physical exercise on some parameters of bone metabolism in postmenopausal women. Endocr Res 1996;22(2):131–8.

Brahm H, Piehl-Aulin K, Ljunghall S, Bone metabolism during exercise and recovery: the influence of plasma volume and physical fitness. Calcif Tissue Int 1997;61(3):192–8.

Van der Wiel HE, Lips P, Graafmans WC, Danielsen CC, Nauta J, van Lingen A, Mosekilde L, Additional weight-bearing during exercise is more important than duration of exercise for anabolic stimulus of bone: a study of running exercise in female rats. Bone 1995;16(1):73–80.

Rong H, Berg U, Trring O, Sundberg CJ, Granberg B, Bucht E, Effects of acute endurance and strength exercise on circulating calcium-regulating hormones and bone markers in young healthy males. Scand J Med Sports 1997;7(3):152–9.

Bourrin S, Palle S, Pupier R, Vico L, Alexandre C, Effect of physical training on bone adaptation in three zones of the rat tibia. J Bone Miner Res 1995;10(11):1745–52.

Kerr D, Morton A, Dick I, Prince R, Exercise effects on bone mass in postmenopausal women are site-specific and load-dependent. J Bone Miner Res 1996;11(2):218–25.

Index

ABOUT THE AUTHORS

Carl Germano, RD, CNS, LDN, is a registered and certified clinical nutritionist and practitioner in Chinese herbology. He holds a masters degree in clinical nutrition from New York University and has over twenty years of experience using innovative, complementary nutritional therapies in private practice. For the past twelve years, he has dedicated his efforts to research and product development for the nutritional supplement industry, where he has been instrumental in bringing cutting-edge nutritional substances and formulations to the market. Presently, he is the vice president of product development with the Solgar Vitamin & Herbs company. Today, he continues his efforts in product development and research and is responsible for providing the health industry with the next generation of clinically important nutritional substances. Mr. Germano is Adjunct Professor of Nutrition at New York Chiropractic College, as well as a frequent radio guest and columnist on the subject of nutrition, and he is coauthor of the best-selling book *The Brain Wellness Plan.*

Dr. William Cabot is an orthopedic surgeon board-certified by the American Board of Orthopedic Surgery and a Fellow of the American Academy of Disability-Evaluating Physicians. Presently, he is President of the William Cabot Group. As an orthopedic surgeon, he was founder of the South Cobb Orthopedic Center and the Southern Back and Orthopedic Center, where he has treated numerous patients with osteoporosis. He has held the position of Chief of Orthopedic Surgery at Emory Adventist Hospital and Cobb General Hospital in Atlanta. Dr. Cabot has numerous publications to his credit and has specialized in the treatment of lower back pain. He is a member of the Board of Directors of Kid's Chance and also served as Clinical Assistant Professor at the Morehouse School of Medicine.